Restoring the Healer

To Jim.

A wonderful physician, and a dear friend & colleague.

Bill

Restoring the Healer

*Spiritual Self-Care
for Health Care Professionals*

William E. Dorman, DMin

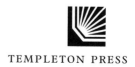

TEMPLETON PRESS

Templeton Press
300 Conshohocken State Road, Suite 500
West Conshohocken, PA 19428
www.templetonpress.org

Designed and typeset by Gopa & Ted2, Inc.

Library of Congress Cataloging-in-Publication Data

Names: Dorman, William E., 1945- , author.
Title: Restoring the healer : spiritual self-care for health care
  professionals / William E. Dorman.
Description: West Conshohocken, PA : Templeton Press, [2015]
Identifiers: LCCN 2015047649 (print) | LCCN 2015049138 (ebook) |
  ISBN 9781599474939 (paperback) | ISBN 9781599474946 (ebook)
Subjects: | MESH: Health Personnel—psychology | Spiritual Therapies-
  methods | Burnout, Professional—prevention & control | Self Care—
  methods | Religion and Psychology | Professional-Patient Relations | Case
  Reports
Classification: LCC BT732.5 (print) | LCC BT732.5 (ebook) | NLM W 21 |
  DDC 615.8/52—dc23
LC record available at http://lccn.loc.gov/2015047649

Printed in the United States of America

16 17 18 19 20   10 9 8 7 6 5 4 3 2 1

For Fran Dorman,
my best friend and soul mate

Contents

Foreword

IN TODAY'S WORLD of deep uncertainty, people are often stressed, questioning the choices they made in their lives and feeling disconnected, unfulfilled, and anxious about what the future might hold. Health care is part of this world and its uncertainties. There are huge changes and challenges in every facet of our clinical professions. Regulations, electronic health records, and packed schedules seem to intrude into the sanctity of the clinician-patient relationship. The complexities of the health system result in clinicians having to help patients navigate system issues that are also complicated for them. At times, the suffering of patients and their families becomes too much for clinicians to bear in the face of an increased workload and system complexities. It is well documented that physician burnout, depression, and suicide are on the rise. Some of the reasons cited are system issues that undermine the physician-patient relationship, the lack of sufficient time to spend with patients in order to provide the best care, and the reductionist medical model that does not honor the humanity of the patient and the clinician. Many clinicians write about needing to be emotionally detached in order to deal with this stress. But for most clinicians, the greatest joy and meaning comes from serving patients. Having to detach in order to "survive" is harmful to the clinician's well-being, for it results in a loss of fulfillment and disconnection from the essence of the vocation. It also results in a distancing from personal wounds and suffering, which leads to greater detachment and burnout.

Where is it, then, that we as clinicians find our healing? It is in the midst of our sacred relationship with our patients: When we sit in silent awe as our patients describe their hope and gratitude in the midst of their struggles with advancing cancer. When we open up to the teachings of our elderly patients who, despite their advanced dementia, share words of profound wisdom. When we celebrate a correct diagnosis and our partnership with our patients in their healing. When at the end of the day we experience gratitude for the privilege we had of entering into relationships, even in small snatches of time, with our patients. It is in those moments that we experience the meaning and the purpose of our lives. And in that instance all is well.

William Dorman's *Restoring the Healer* offers the insight and resources for all clinicians to reconnect with their call to be healers. He shows us how to find awe again in the healing encounters with our patients. He inspires us to infuse our reductionist medical model with humanity, spirituality, and compassion. He helps us touch the wounded healer within and gently restores us to openness to the mystery of all we do, even in the midst of professional uncertainty and stress. He helps us recapture our enthusiasm—the enthusiasm we all had when we decided to enter the healing professions—to be present to others and to make a difference in the lives of all the patients we serve.

Christina M. Puchalski, MD

Preface

YOU HAVE COMMITTED your life to the well-being of others. You offer hope and encouragement to your patients, in addition to providing care. This book is an appreciation of the profound difference you make and an acknowledgement of the stress you experience in your efforts as a healer. That's why I am convinced that *your* self-care is equally important to the well-being of your patients. If you are not well, how can you serve your community? At its heart, this book is directed toward your well-being. My sincere hope is that it offers insights that you will find both illuminating and rewarding, and that it will help you heal.

During your education and training, you were introduced to the concept of spirituality within the context of health care. It is common today for health care professionals to see physical health as encompassing body, mind, and spirit. Spirituality is a vital factor in human well-being. And yet, it is typically reserved for end-of-life care, cultural diversity, and the treatment choices a patient makes based on his or her religious or spiritual beliefs.

However, my understanding of spirituality is broadly based and ecumenical. It is grounded in the basic human experience of wonder and awe. Such experience-based spirituality is a natural outgrowth of simple, child-like fascination. Perhaps you occasionally experience moments of amazement when you marvel at the intricacy, delicacy, and complexity of human well-being. You experience life's beginning and end, its meaning and purpose, and its possibilities and limits. Spirituality and science have one essential ingredient in common: experience as the basis of wonder and awe. Perhaps your fascination with the wellsprings of life is what initially inspired you to devote yourself to such a demanding profession.

So this book is not about patients per se: it is about you. As a caregiver, you are trained to focus exclusively on your patients. The unique perspective offered here shifts that focus to your emotional and spiritual well-being as well. In the process, both you and your patients can benefit greatly.

Central to your professional identity is your confidence in your knowledge and skills. You value being perceived as clear-headed, decisive, and steady. It is important that you keep your professional persona intact so that your colleagues see that you are able to take the heat in the kitchen. There can be a not-so-subtle pride among health care professionals about being able to handle whatever comes their way, and to move onto the next patient or case without blinking an eye. Bravado is instilled in you as part of your training and socialization as a health care professional. Certain teams and disciplines pride themselves on being able to jump from one crisis to the next. But make no mistake, practicing spiritual self-care is not a weakness: it is a strength.

It is quite possible that you grasp the importance of self-care but wonder, "Where in the world will I fit one more thing into my busy day?" This book respects the demands on your time and suggests ways in which you can practice self-care as you go about your patient care. Self-care is not indulgent. It is not another thing added to your already busy day. It is (or can be) an integral part of it.

Call to mind those times when you were a patient: having a routine checkup; making an appointment because you noticed something you thought merited attention; ending up in the emergency room following an automobile accident. In those moments, you were the patient. Your well-being was the primary focus. Granted, this role may have made you uncomfortable. And yet, you may have experienced some degree of gratitude for the care you received during those moments. It is my hope that this book will stir a similar gratitude for the care it extends to you.

I realize and respect the apprehension among health care professionals when it comes to personal feelings and emotions. Your worries about work or home are best kept confidential. You are in a culture where the expression of second thoughts—worry, frustration, or despondency—is not encouraged. You want to appear self-confident, dispassionate, and unflappable. Health care professionals who are troubled by professional or personal situations seek confidential help—if they seek help at all. It might be said that health care professionals hide emotions and feelings because of a culture of secrecy.

This culture can lead to unwelcome outcomes. You may become anxious, fretful, withdrawn, or irritable. You may develop headaches, tight shoulder or neck muscles, or an upset stomach. You may turn to substances—controlled and over-the-counter—to help you get through the day. This book offers a healthy alternative to self-destructive behaviors.

It seems to me that the conversation in recent books and journals about *compassion fatigue* hints at a growing willingness among health care professionals to consider their own well-being. What you experience may be more aptly called *caring fatigue*, a phenomenon inclusive of the drain on your body, mind, and spirit. The self-care aspect of this book directly addresses this situation, offering you insights about how to take care of yourself. It's intended to be both preventative as well as restorative in nature.

I hope my initial comments speak to your heart and mind. Maybe these few words resemble an *informed consent* of sorts, one that provides you a better idea of the nature of this book, which is to offer you healing. It is my hope that you will allow us to continue this conversation in the following pages.

You may be wondering, "Why you? Who are you to dispense this sort of counsel?" This book rests on my eighteen years of experience working as a board certified professional chaplain in the anchor hospital of an integrated health care system. The system included hospitals in town and across the state, a physicians' medical group, and a health plan. At that time, the downtown hospital was one among several major hospitals in the community.

When I began my work, I was assigned to all the critical care units in both the organization's community hospital and the downtown hospital. These units consisted of the following: a cardiac critical care unit and an adult intensive care unit at the community hospital and a cardiac critical care unit, an adult intensive care unit, a subacute care unit, a neonatal intensive care unit, and a pediatric intensive care unit at the downtown facility. I made routine rounds on these units, carrying a pager to respond to requests for a chaplain. In addition, I was involved in overnight, in-house on-calls, during which time I was the only chaplain available.

I had two other major roles during my time as a professional chaplain: I served on the Hospital Ethics Committee (HEC) and the Crisis Support Team. Along with the HEC chair and the HEC coordinator, I helped plan the agenda for the monthly meetings and held a key role in responding to requests for ethics consults. I assisted in setting up the ethics consults and routinely participated in them. The Crisis Support Team provided critical incident stress management support to the clinicians, staff, and employees throughout the organization. I had a leadership role in this team and also served as a responder to support individuals and/or teams experiencing a trauma.

True to the experience-based foundation of the book, what I write about is rooted in my time spent working in the hospital. That included the spiritual care and emotional support of patients, families, and staff. In this book, I have drawn from these experiences but masked and disguised them in order to preserve and protect privacy and confidentiality. These accounts capture the spiritual and emotional stress involved in healing, highlighting the importance of spirituality and self-care for the healers' own well-being.

As a chaplain, I witnessed the toll and drain experienced by health care professionals, such as:

▸ Physicians and nurses delivering a premature fetus, and gently and compassionately handing the body to the mother to be cradled.

▸ First responders transferring a teenager who had attempted suicide to the emergency room team, standing by anxiously to await the outcome. Outside the treatment room, the teenager's parents waited in anguished silence, holding on to hope for their child.

▸ A nurse somberly entering the room of a dying patient, and with tears in her eyes, administering morphine to ease the patient's terminal breathing.

▸ Physicians expressing their inner turmoil over a patient's family's request for an intervention that offered no benefit and sought no treatment goal, serving only to subject the patient to invasive and painful procedures.

▸ Nurses and physicians sitting in the break room one morning, reflecting on the unexpected "limp baby" they had delivered and quickly rushed to the neonatal intensive care unit.

▸ A physician meeting with sad and worried family members, hoping to explain compassionately that a do not resuscitate (DNR) order would allow for a peaceful and dignified death for their dying loved one and avoid the invasive efforts of resuscitation required without the order in place.

▸ Nurses and physicians standing in disbelief and grief at a nurses' station as they heard the news of their colleague's successful suicide.

▸ A team struggling with their anger and sorrow at the betrayal and dishonesty of one of their team members who had been caught diverting drugs.

These incidents stirred in me a realization of the emotional and spiritual impact absorbed by health care professionals as they go about their healing tasks. These experiences are this book's bedrock, and they are the inspiration for my commitment to the health care professional's well-being. My goal for this book is to provide spiritual resources and self-care insights that will help healers be more resilient and give them methods for cultivating a deep and lasting satisfaction with their healing careers.

Acknowledgments

FOR YEARS I had the idea to write a book on spirituality and health care. During a lunch conversation, William H. Brady III, MD, and Shar Haley, RN, encouraged me to write the book, providing me with insights, resources, and direction from their writing experiences. Over the span of two years, I gave drafts of chapters to friends and colleagues, asking for their critique and recommendations. I am grateful to James M. Gustafson, PhD; Paul Hopkins, DMin; Jimmy Hood, PhD; Diane J. Sansonetti, MD; Shar Haley, RN, and William H. Brady III, MD, for their helpful comments. I am indebted to Meg Ashcroft, my spiritual director, for her encouragement.

I thank the staff at Templeton Press: Susan Arellano, publisher; Angelina Horst, editorial and social media content coordinator; and Trish Vergilio, production manager. They have worked with me from the beginning of this project. Karen Kelly's editing skills helped hone the book. *Restoring the Healer* would not have become a reality without them.

I am most appreciative to my wife, Fran Dorman. Fran is a physical therapist with years of experience in health care as a clinician and an administrator. She has been my primary source of encouragement and my chief editor. She patiently read the manuscript as it evolved, keeping me on track with her insightful questions and suggestions.

Restoring the Healer

Introduction

THIS BOOK OFFERS healing to healers. It is experience based. Actual experience in a hospital is the anvil upon which this book has been hammered and fashioned.

Your career began with your training, where you were introduced to the educational model known as *problem-based learning*, an experience-based approach. Once you completed your education, you began practice as a healer, over time becoming an experienced health care professional. With every interaction with patients and their families, you draw upon the vast reservoir of knowledge you have acquired. This experience guides you through the day as you encounter both the familiar and the novel.

Spirituality is likewise experience based, specifically encountering wonder and awe, the origin of human spirituality. In moments of wonder and awe, we experience the Transcendent Source of Life, which is the awareness of those powers beyond us that provide limits as well as possibilities. These times call forth from us the senses of gratitude, interdependence, purpose, and humility. Throughout the book, I draw on these dimensions of human spirituality to show how spirituality benefits you professionally and personally. I am indebted to my friend and colleague James M. Gustafson, PhD, author of *Ethics from a Theocentric Perspective,*

Volumes I and II, for my understanding of spirituality as experience based, and of the resultant senses.

Health care occurs through the coordinated efforts of a vast network of people. Certainly those directly involved in patient care come to mind—physicians, advanced practice clinicians, nurses, techs, aides, chaplains, social workers, and therapists (physical therapists, occupational therapists, respiratory therapists, behavioral health therapists). These healers are the more visible members of this vast network.

In addition, there is an extensive and less-visible network essential to providing health care: accounting, pharmacy, housekeeping, quality improvement, security, dietary, maintenance, research, legal services, risk management, continuing education, medical library, compliance, infection control, purchasing, safety, shipping and receiving, disaster planning, human resources, operations, real estate, leadership, boards, committees, information technology, and more. Mindful of the indispensable role each individual and every team plays in delivering quality health care, my focus is largely on those who provide direct care and service to patients and families in the hospital setting (i.e., physicians, advanced practice clinicians, and nurses).

Health care is a wonderful and difficult world. Putting aside all the policies, regulations, and laws of health care, it involves some of the most poignant and touching moments and experiences imaginable. These may be as subtle as the moving inflection of a few words or as graphic as a complicated and threatened pregnancy resolving in a successful delivery—healthy baby, healthy mom.

Some of you reading this book may already be enrolled in professional schools: medical, nursing, physical therapy, occupational therapy, pharmacy, respiratory therapy, divinity, mental health. Some of you may be considering a career in health care. In that light, this book will provide you snapshots of what it is like to be a health care professional. Still some of you may be members of the general public, including former and current patients. And yet others of you may presently lack direct contact with hospital-based care, but are curious and interested in that world.

In today's climate of radical changes, looming challenges, and promising advances in health care, there is a widespread interest in "taking a peek" into the world of health care. What is it like to be a patient? Who are these professionals to whom the public turns to in times of need?

I suspect that a majority of you reading this book are health care professionals. You are already engaged in healing as a physician, advanced practice clinician, or nurse. You know firsthand the privilege of being invited by patients and their families to participate in life's most intimate and moving interactions and experiences. In this sacred arena, lives are saved—or lost. Babies are born. Tears of joy and sorrow are shed. Sighs of despair and sighs of relief escape people's mouths. Words of anger flash like lightning. While monitors blink and ventilators hiss, silence stills the room. Wailing rises and falls. Emotions are bared, and bodies are naked. Life comes down to days, hours, minutes, and seconds. The question, "What is the meaning of all this?" enters the minds of patients, family, and health care team members. What is of value and importance may be adjusted, abandoned, or affirmed. Anxiety, peace, fear, courage, suffering of body and soul, kindness, dignity, tragedy, beauty, and horror come and go as waves on the beach.

Some of your days are routine. On occasion, there may be a

lull, even a hint of boring inactivity. At other times, you are caught up in a surge of tremendous intensity and electrifying stress. Stable patients suddenly and unexpectedly crash. Struggling patients amazingly turn the corner for the better. You have days of deep professional pride and satisfaction. Other days are disheartening and disconcerting to you personally and professionally. Health care is grueling and gratifying. What an amazing and astounding world!

You certainly know the apprehension, anxiety, ambiguity, and uncertainty generated by the major changes underway in health care. The Affordable Care Act is making fundamental alterations to how health care is accessed, provided, and funded. Accompanying the changes required by the Affordable Care Act are the concurrent changes in Medicare and Medicaid. The Centers for Medicare & Medicaid Services (CMS) are introducing and implementing changes in what health conditions and treatments are covered and implementing reimbursement changes that affect patients, providers, health care plans, and health care organizations.

In today's stormy sea of drastic change, health care workers are quite worried, even anxious. As a healer, you have invested your life in the pursuit of your role. You have expended significant amounts of time and money to acquire the training and experience to qualify for your position. You wonder what will become of you individually. Is there a place for you in health care given today's climate and circumstances? How do you plan for the future, since the continuing stops and starts within health care make it increasingly difficult to plan for today, let alone for tomorrow? Simply facing today's expectations is no small task, and it can be even more difficult to look ahead to your career path.

Documentation is becoming more and more time consuming, expensive, and complex. Yes, the Electronic Medical Record (EMR) is being launched amid much applause. However, you continue to swim in a sea of paper. Though the shift is to electronic documentation, the information still has to be entered into the patient record (database). Whether the documentation is paper or electronic, you must devote time to it. Time spent with records and documentation takes time away from your passion (i.e., patients). The actual value of the EMR is fast and easy access to a patient's medical records, promising improvements in patient safety and the quality of patient care. There is no doubt that achieving these values is intensive in both time and capital. And the burden of dealing with these changes falls on you, the health care provider.

This book is offered as a gift. It bestows to you, as a health care professional, a breath of fresh air. You will discover a momentary oasis, with these pages serving as a soul spa where you are able to reflect and reenergize. I invite you to a peaceful and sacred space, a space to be found in the parking lot, the nurses' station, the staff break room, or the hospital chapel. This space is not limited to physical locales: it is frequently a virtual space, one residing in the recesses of your heart and soul. This inward journey prepares you to move outward into the hallowed halls of healing.

How to Use This Book

Generally speaking, readers approach a book intending to read it from beginning to end. You can certainly elect to read this book in that fashion, especially when coming to it for the first time. I have also written and formatted *Restoring the Healer* to encourage browsing, so you can self-select the order in which you read it. Each of the chapters contains a narrative, patient stories, and a concluding section of prayers, meditations, and reflections, all addressing the topic of that chapter. A scan of the table of contents gives a clear picture of the topics covered, and one of them may address an issue you are confronting at the moment. Feel free to go directly to chapters that draw you in.

I also suggest that you take time to absorb the chapters as you read them, before rushing on to the next. There is value in pausing to digest the sections of this book that resonate with you. When these moments come, spend time with the thoughts and feelings you experience. One value of patient stories is the awareness and affirmation that other health care professionals—your colleagues—have similar experiences, thoughts, and feelings.

The prayers, meditations, reflections, and rituals in each chapter are specifically meant to offer an opportunity to pause and be still. These resources are intended for your ongoing use as you customize and integrate them into your day. Accept the book's invitation to spend a few moments of quiet and rest.

Restoring the Healer intends to be a resource for you, so you may view it as a different kind of caregiver's manual, one that is centered on *your* needs. You already have electronic and printed manuals at your fingertips, all of which pertain to patient care. This manual pertains to your self-care and to your well-being. I hope that you dog-ear, highlight, and bookmark those sections that speak to you.

CHAPTER I

Embrace Awe

THE MORE YOU ARE able to pay attention to your world, the more you will behold marvels. Wonder is an everyday experience. A good number of instances of wonder are quite ordinary and might go unappreciated—even unrecognized. Some of these experiences are of a larger scale and are of such dimensions that it is hard for them to escape notice or be dismissed. In either case—from the small to the sizeable—being attentive is the window through which we behold such moments. These experiences are the primary basis for spirituality. In such times, we discover the Transcendent Source of Life and find our lives reshaped and redirected.

Awe offers you an opportunity to sense mysteries beyond your comprehension. It speaks of the unknown and touches you in your depths, moving you to moments of deep contemplation and reflection on this mystery we call life.

Whether a person's response to wonder and awe evokes a religious (spiritual) or philosophical response, fascination is alive and well in the hearts and souls of all who gaze upon the beauty, intricacy, expanse, and depth of life. What follows is an amazing story of a "just in time" discovery.

JOHN'S STORY: ROUTINE MIRACLES

John had been scheduled for a routine surgery, a hernia repair. During the requisite presurgery workups, doctors discovered an aortic aneurism. The health care team moved into high gear. John and his family were informed of the aneurism and the need for immediate surgery to correct this life-threatening situation. With John's consent, he was taken to the presurgery area to be prepared for the new procedure.

Without the need for the hernia repair, the aneurism on his aorta would have continued to remain an undetected condition, one with the potential to end John's life suddenly and unexpectedly. John and his family were relieved and grateful that this threat had been identified and corrected. It was a moment of wonder and gratitude for them.

It is beyond knowing how John's aneurism remained intact until he scheduled his hernia repair. This one instance can be multiplied as you recall similar such moments of unknown reasons.

Healers are drawn to health care by its myriad wonders. You are intrigued with the human being—muscles, nerves, joints, organs, biology, chemistry, cells, wellness, disease, emotions, thoughts, and therapies. Through the course of your training, wonder may prompt you to focus on one aspect of human well-being, which you choose as your specialty or subspecialty. Some healers concentrate on an organ or system: lungs, kidneys, or hearts. Others develop an interest in patient populations: newborns, cancer, aging, diabetics, closed head injuries, spinal cord injuries, amputees, or behavioral health. No matter your specialty, you are filled with a hunger to know more so that you may improve the well-being of those patients who require help from your field of health care.

Your efforts to help your patients achieve wellness succeed to varying degrees. You see some patients achieve a complete restoration of their health. These patients are able to resume their lives. At other times, you encounter those patients for whom you and your colleagues are able to provide little if any improvement in their health status.

Let's take a look at a situation where the entire interdisciplinary team was frustrated. They were stumped. No matter how much they wanted to help the patient, their efforts failed. The mood was one of discouragement. There was general knowledge about how this case would play out—and that the outcome would be a sad one. There appeared to be little if any reason for wonder in the situation.

JOANNA'S STORY: THE GIFT OF BREATHING

Regardless of the critical care unit team's best efforts, they were unable to wean Joanna from the ventilator. The patient's mother was beside herself with worry for her daughter. The team held consultations with specialists and subspecialists from within and from beyond the hospital. At every turn, they reached a dead end. The team held several ethics consults with Joanna's family (the patient lacked capacity and her family members were her decision-makers), describing the risks and benefits as they explored treatment options. The dilemma was that the trach tube had to be removed. It had been inserted in the patient's airway for such a lengthy period of time that the health care team was concerned that the treatment itself posed a great risk to the patient.

Finally, it was agreed that Joanna would be extubated. The team explained to the patient's mother that her daughter may take no breath, a few breaths, or breathe for an hour or two, perhaps two days at most. There was a slim possibility that she would resume breathing on her own, but the previous failed weaning efforts gave little to no reason to think the patient could breathe independently.

The health care team removed the tube with the mother and other family members gathered at the bedside. The patient began to breathe. The team cautioned the mother not to pin too much hope on these early and feeble breaths. Minutes stretched into hours, and then hours stretched to the end of day one. On day two, Joanna continued to breathe on her own and appeared to be getting stronger. By the end of the week, she was breathing independently and was discharged home.

What happened? How was this resumption of breathing possible? Where did Joanna get the strength to breathe on her own after being on a ventilator so long? What the team witnessed was beyond explanation. It flew in the face of reason. No one could have predicted this outcome—and no one did! To the contrary, the family and the critical care team were resolved to what seemed to be the inescapable conclusion of this saga—the patient's death. However, discouragement and disillusionment were banished by amazement. Joanna's breathing gratefully astounded the family and the health care team.

Generally, you are able to predict, or prognosticate, the course and end of a case. Many times, you wish what was ahead for the patient was not so and that you could affect a different outcome. Every so often, what you do not expect, thankfully, is precisely what happens.

DAVID'S STORY: UNTANGLED KNOTS

David was admitted to the hospital complaining of severe abdominal pain. After a prompt and thorough workup, the doctors informed David that he had a bowel obstruction. The bowel had somehow developed a twist that blocked the bowel. The health care team recommended a surgery to correct this potentially life-threatening problem. Before the surgery could be performed, the obstruction unexpectedly resolved. The bowel "righted itself" and resumed normal function.

There are rare reports of such spontaneous resolution. Certainly, David and his family were relieved when the physician delivered the wonderful news! Their somber moods were replaced by marvel and gratitude.

Such moments of spontaneous resolution fill you with astonishment at the depths and mysteries of life. You wonder at the incredible resiliency demonstrated by some patients. These moments of the incredible offer you joy and gratitude, because sometimes you do not know the full story. It is important for you to maintain a certain professional and experienced uncertainty, an uncertainty that is honed on the sharpening wheel of past cases. More often than not, your prognosis is on target. However, there are those rare instances where the diagnosis and prognosis prove not to be accurate that help you preserve a small amount of respect and reservation for the fact that cases do not always turn out as anticipated or projected.

These times are opportunities for you to develop your disposition of humility. More will be said about humility in chapter 11. During this present discussion of wonder and awe, it is worth noting that humility is close by when you experience wonder. The two cases discussed earlier—Joanna's extubation and David's bowl obstruction—ended on a note of gratitude. You fully know that the opposite outcome is equally possible. There are those patient care moments when a positive outcome is reasonably expected. Those expectations may be shattered by a tragic, or at best, a limited outcome. In these instances, the wonder does not lead to gratitude, but to sorrow.

Eric's Story: "I'm Outta Here!"

Eric was a homeless male who came to the emergency room complaining about a cut on his forearm. What had begun as a small cut on his arm had developed into a wound with a raging infection, threatening his limb and life. Once Eric was admitted to the hospital, the health care team diagnosed the infection and began to administer the appropriate antibiotic intravenously. The antibiotic was effective, and the infection began to recede.

Feeling better, Eric stated that he wanted to leave the hospital. The health care team attempted to communicate the seriousness of his condition and the importance of completing his antibiotic treatment. In spite of the health care team's efforts to describe graphically the dire consequences of leaving the hospital, Eric was adamant about leaving.

Given his determination, the health care team presented him the "against medical advice" discharge papers. He signed the papers and left the hospital. The health care team was astonished. The patient's decision mystified them. They wondered what was so important to the patient about leaving the hospital that he was willing to put his life at severe risk. They were also left wondering about their ineffective efforts to persuade Eric to stay in the hospital.

The above clinical example is an instance of sorrowful wonder. The episode portrays those times when there are circumstances beyond the influence, and certainly the control, of the health care team. Reasoned conversation, generally effective in discussing treatment options and the accompanying risks and benefits, proved ineffective in this situation. The involved healers were both sad and perplexed.

Prayers, Meditations, and Reflections

Constancy and Wonder

⊐ Center of Constancy, I stand astounded at the predictability of life. Healing is built upon outcomes and upon replication. Constancy is not dulling—it is fascinating! May I always marvel at the way I can count on sameness. When the unusual, the anomaly, does appear, help me to be unafraid—not to be dismayed, but to be intrigued. For the beauty and wonder filling each day, I give you thanks. Especially, I thank you for my eyes, my mind, my heart, my soul—all of which are portals of amazement. Amen.

The Unexpected

Rainbow-Maker, your colorful spectrum illumines my horizon. Against my fixed horizon of constancy and routine, you cast your unexpected light show on the screens of dark clouds. Thank you for this sacred gift of wonder as I gaze upon the incredible. How can color come from such grayness? Where else in my life are rainbows gleaming, waiting for my attentive eye? While I value routine, I hunger for the color and light of the unexpected in life, those rainbow moments when I see as I never saw before. Amen.

When Things Fall Short

World-Maker, do unexpected things happen to you? Not a welcome surprise, but a shocking turn of events? Do you ever wish that some hurricanes and earthquakes were not so horrendous? Do you shrink back from the brutality that humans inflict upon one another and the planet? Did you see that coming?

I find myself dismayed, not wondering. I am in shock. I am incredulous at how the patient who was doing so well suddenly took a nosedive! I am angry, disappointed, and sad.

Unwelcome and unforeseen outcomes do appear, which in hindsight are clearer to the eye. These unexpected consequences dare me to explain how I failed to take them into consideration. Free me from hindsight's painful grip.

Transform my self-berating into humility. Neither my colleagues nor I are all knowing. Help me to gain perspective on this event so that in the face of the ever-present unforeseen, I continue to be a wise and prudent healer. Amen.

Journaling

A journal is a beneficial way to meditate on the day. Writing down your thoughts puts them before you on the page, where you are able to see them. Looking at what you write permits you to gaze into your heart and soul. Let your writing be as free flowing as possible, with little—if any—self-censure. You will find a healing and a peace in getting your thoughts and feelings out of your head and heart and onto a piece of paper where they are less distressing. Your journaling creates a vista from which you are able to look down into your life's valleys, look back to where you have been, look up to life's peaks, or to look ahead into the indistinct, yet discernible, future.

Lighting a Candle

The practical value of candles has largely been lost given the modern forms of light. Apart from the power of illumination, candles continue to offer another value, that of creating a peaceful and fascinating setting. Places of worship, personal shrines at home, public shrines prompted by a community sorrow, and places where meals are served all continue to honor the value of a candle to create a certain mood.

Candles are a simple means by which you can pause, be still, and reflect. There is a ritual in the lighting of the candle (or candles) itself. After lighting the candle, let it draw you into its world of dancing light and flickering brilliance. A candle offers silence—a rare gift in today's world. It offers no image, but beckons your heart and soul to bring forth their pictures for you to behold in your mind's eye.

Light a candle. Sit back. Gaze upon it. Be silent. Be still. You will be soothed.

CHAPTER 2

Heal Your Inner Healer

WHAT IS *spirituality?* The word is widely used and has certainly become part of the parlance within health care itself. Given its diverse and frequent appearance in conversation—written and spoken—it has multiple definitions. As a matter of fact, it has so many uses and definitions that the term is diluted, lacking the power of depth and precision required to be of benefit to conversation and thought.

Here is my definition: "Spirituality is a human's capacity to experience the Transcendent Source of Life that envelopes and nurtures all creation, offers possibilities while setting limits, and evokes a sense of awe, gratitude, interdependence, direction, obligation, accountability, and humility." (I have adapted this definition with permission from *Ethics from a Theocentric Perspective, Volumes I and II* by James M. Gustafson, PhD.)

In the early pages of this book, I stated that this book is experiential, not theoretical. My goal is to talk with you in terms of experience, not theory. I referenced problem-based learning earlier as the key modality for describing spirituality and dialoguing about it. Spirituality is experiential. Previously, I commented that the primary experience of spirituality are moments of wonder and awe. Spirituality arises from that foundational occurrence. The patient care example that follows provides a specific instance of wonder and awe.

MARY'S STORY: FINAL BLESSING

The scene in the intensive care unit room was tragic. A young mother was dying of cirrhosis of the liver, a condition caused by years of heavy alcohol consumption. Gathered around her bed were her mother, her sister, and her two school-age sons. Mary's family was sobbing, their hearts broken. As the patient's breaths came fewer and farther apart, her mother and sister began to sing. Their singing was spontaneous, a calling to mind of a then-popular song. The song was dirge-like, a soulful mourning, their voices a muted wail. Yet, the lyrics brought hope and healing to the room. Mary's sad life was acknowledged, but her mother and sister were blessing her, singing a prayer that finally her life would know peace and fulfillment. Those members of the health care team standing in the room with the family, and those gathered in the doorway, were spellbound.

There was no doubt that Mary's life had been tortured. She had known abuse, neglect, rejection, and failed relationships. The alcohol she had turned to in search of comfort and courage had turned on her, claiming her life. Mary's mother's heart was broken for her child who never saw the simple joys of life. Yet, at her daughter's bedside, she was able to sing a song of sorrow and of blessing for this child of hers.

It was a moment of wonder! No words of reprimand were spoken. No anger was expressed. Words of love and encouragement bathed the patient in her last moments. The action of Mary's mother and sister showed enormous resiliency, courage, and creativity. Their singing and presence transformed that intensive care unit room into a sacred space of grace, forgiveness, and hope. How is that possible in the presence of such tragedy?

It is quite possible to find this episode empty of wonder. It may be viewed as common, even predictable. Those in health care know that sobbing family members often stand by the bed of a loved one dying from alcohol-induced cirrhosis of the liver. The family is sad and frustrated, resigned to the fate that awaited their loved one all along, who, despite all their efforts, continued to consume alcohol in devastating amounts.

It is precisely these multiple other instances of resignation that make Mary's story such an amazing contrast. In this particular experience, the patient's mother and sister transformed a tragic moment into a moment of grace and blessing. This distinctiveness is precisely the cause for wonder.

This case is an experience. It makes an impact on the observers, transforming them into participants as the event engages and interacts with them. The intensive care unit event was an experience stretched over time, comprised of people—patient, family, and healers—moving step-by-step as death escorted life from the room.

In this clinical episode, we discern that beneath the surface and appearances of life, there is an immense and wonderful depth: joy, ideas, beauty, sorrow, kindness, devotion, love, and connection. These experiences are all entry points of the spiritual into our lives.

You have had those experiences where the patient responds in a unique and amazing manner to his or her plight. These patients are quite aware of the gravity of their disease or injury, and certainly exhibit signs of the shock and physical pain that they are undergoing.

At the same time, these patients, who are ordinary people and who come from all walks of life, demonstrate a remarkable resiliency. Somehow, from deep within their heart and soul, they draw upon strengths that prevent such traumatic occurrences from dominating, devastating, or overwhelming them. What follows is an illustration of just such an attribute exhibited by an elderly female.

Evelyn's Story: Perseverance Personified

When the elderly female patient arrived in the emergency department and was transported from the ambulance to the treatment room, what the team saw shocked them. Evelyn was a bloody, gory mess. Her fragile skin was torn, with sheets of skin hanging from her extremities. She had been relentlessly raped and beaten over a lengthy period of time. The emergency department team moved quickly to assess and stabilize her. It became clear that her injuries were not life threatening and that she would survive this savage attack.

Once she was stabilized, the nurses began to clean and treat her multiple wounds. Those nurses assigned to this task spent their entire shift (12 hours) caring for this elderly victim of rape and battery.

After Evelyn's wounds were attended, and the requisite sexual assault questions and examinations completed, the patient was transferred to a hospital floor. Her family had been present the entire time and accompanied her to her room, where they surrounded her with comfort and love.

In sharp contrast to the trauma she had undergone, what the health care team witnessed and experienced was her astounding resiliency. This lady possessed remarkable stamina and an unrelenting positive attitude. Where one might reasonably expect anxiety, if not resentment, she was even-keeled. Foremost on Evelyn's mind was the intent of regaining her health and strength so that she could return to her apartment where she lived independently. Getting home to her apartment and friends—that was her goal. She was aware that she had been brutalized and could have died. But what mattered to her was the kindness of the staff and the support of her family and friends. Evelyn was grateful for the care she was receiving and grateful to be alive.

Whenever the staff entered her room, they experienced a hopeful, courageous woman. She made it clear that what had happened was not going to get the best of her. The staff was in awe of her stamina of body, mind, and spirit. They marveled at how Evelyn was able to put this tragedy into perspective. Her sense of humor was inspirational and lifted the spirits of the staff. Going into Evelyn's room was healing for the healers. How did she do that?

Patients like Evelyn, who in the midst of an illness or injury maintain a positive attitude, a cheerful demeanor, and a resolve to recover and return to their lives, are a sacred gift to those who are fortunate enough to come into contact with them. It is accurate to describe such patients as a blessing. You are grateful to enter that room and talk with the patient. You find these patients uplifting.

These patients are like manna in the desert during your bleak and tiresome days. They energize you. They nurture your heart and soul. In the years to come, you will draw inspiration, stamina, and encouragement from your memories of these patients. Healers share an old adage: "I get more from that patient than I am able to give him or her." These patients are examples of what matters in life. They renew the compassion, care, and energy required to push ahead on your path as a healer. When you encounter such patients, be grateful and receptive to the gifts they offer you. Many a time—not always, but on occasion—it will happen that you experience a healer-patient relationship that deepens your soul, touches your heart, and lifts your spirit.

Still, moments come when humans are aware (this awareness is a spiritual experience) that there are those forces and powers beyond us and greater than we (economics, politics, injury, disease, human finitude, nature, to name a few). These powers transcend human abilities. These forces envelope, or contain, human effort. In health care, this moment of experiencing what is more powerful than human ability is another form of experiencing the Transcendent Source of Life.

This element of the Transcendent Source of Life, both to set limits and provide possibilities, is portrayed in the following instance. At one point in the case, there seemed to be quite reasonable and attainable possibilities. Then, as health care moved along, the limits of the situation sadly became more and more evident.

RACHEL'S STORY: SOMETIMES IT HURTS

The patient and the healers knew that it was an uphill battle, but they saw a chance that the cancer could be overcome. Optimism was in the air. Rachel was a young, healthy female. She was a single parent with children at home who was supported and encouraged by a large circle of family and friends. She had surgery, followed by subsequent regimens of chemotherapy and radiation. The cancer was in remission, and she was doing well. In light of her progress, she was transferred to a rehabilitation program and began to recover her strength. Both the patient and healers were confident as she quickly progressed. However, the disease reappeared, and once again she began chemotherapy. Every week, Rachel came for her treatment at the cancer center. During her time in the hospital, the rehabilitation center, and the infusion center, she and her health care team developed genuine friendships. The staff cared deeply for this patient and wanted her to do well. They felt keenly that this patient and her situation were in their hands—that they had a grip on this case.

Her clinical situation began to decline. Rachel was losing weight and becoming progressively weaker. Diagnostics revealed that the cancer was spreading. Her body was wearing out, and medicine had exhausted its healing capabilities. The limits of what was possible for her had been reached. She was slipping through the health care team's fingers.

The next step was clear to everyone: the decision was made for her to enter hospice care so that Rachel could be at home, where she could be comfortable. Her death was peaceful. Her family and friends surrounded her. When the news of her death reached the staff at the hospital, cancer center, and rehabilitation unit, the healers were profoundly saddened. Rachel's death was a great personal and professional loss to them.

This case is a somber reminder of what you already know: we as humans, and you as a healer, are limited in knowledge and ability. In the above case, the health care team employed best practices.

The team followed standards of care rigorously. The healers and the patient had a high level of confidence that her disease could be managed with a great degree of success.

This patient was stalwart and robust, and her varied treatments did slow the disease. Nonetheless, in the course of her treatment, the limits of the human body itself could be seen as the disease exacted its toll on her body, mind, and spirit. Added to the debilitating effects of the disease itself was the strain accompanying the surgery, chemotherapy, and radiation treatment. Medicine itself, as powerful and advanced as were the interventions administered to improve her health, drew from its well of resources until that well ran dry.

PRAYERS, MEDITATIONS, AND REFLECTIONS

Reality Redefined

Holy Healer, I want you to know that my world is quite empirical. What is real to me is what I can measure. Well, at least, that is what I used to think. Measurement is vital in being a good healer. What I have discovered is that there are immeasurable realities in life—love, hope, uncertainty, fear, sadness, courage, resiliency. Surprisingly, I have learned how to measure these elements! I see it in facial expressions, elevated or decreased respiration or heart rate, optimism, determination. Thank you for broadening my horizons of reality. Amen.

Sometimes Things Drop into Your Lap

Wellspring of Wonders, I guess I could be angry at myself for being stumped. Or I could chastise myself for my inadequacies. Anger and self-abasement ill serve me with their fruits of discouragement and self-doubt. Open my heart and mind to gratitude that a colleague mentioned a similar case in which a certain course benefited that patient. Help me view with wonder that my chance reading of a journal article helped me see new possibilities. Rather than belittle myself when I come to an impasse, help me to be grateful that sometimes things simply drop into my lap. Thank you. Amen.

Not What I Want, but What Is Best for the Patient

I confess, Granter of Goodness, that I have a personal and professional investment in this patient's well-being. My patient is a good person. Her family adores her, and her friends admire her. She deserves more life. She trusts me and has valiantly cooperated in her care. I see the test results. I see the fatigue and the pain in her face and eyes. Clinically, I know that the time is at hand to emphasize quality of life—finding comfort, being with family, and enjoying what brings her delight. Grant me the compassion to put her well-being above my own needs to succeed. Help me to see that my succeeding is to be found to the extent I help this patient achieve her preferences and wishes. It is her life. I am her servant. Amen.

Easy Exercises for Wonder

1. **Sight:** Take a moment to watch the sun rise or the sun set as you begin or end your day. Attend to the colors, patterns, light, and horizon. See if you can experience

fascination at such a magnificent and daily event. Ponder the amazing gift of sight—isn't the eye in itself a marvel?

2. **Sound:** Listen to music. Select music you like. Play it at home, in your car as you commute or run errands, or as you exercise. Listen to the notes, the chords, the instruments, the voice(s), and the rhythm. Music is fascinating, being shaped by genre, culture, influences, and period. See if you can let the music carry you where it will take you. Contemplate sound: both the physics as well as the pitch. Consider how the gift of hearing enriches your life at so many points.

3. **Motion:** Put on your work attire—suit, uniform, shoes, scrubs. Feel your fingers pulling zippers and working with buttons or snaps. Focus on the coordinated movement of your hands, arms, legs, and feet. The agility and intricacy of your body's movement are astounding—muscles, nerves, brain, spinal cord, and the sense of balance all orchestrating fingers, limbs, and trunk. Be amazed at the astonishing abilities of your body. (Walking or exercising provides you with additional moments to be amazed at your body's ability to move.)

4. **Taste:** Drink your favorite beverage or take a bite of your favorite morning dish. Let the taste linger on your palate. Feel the warmth or coolness of the beverage. Focus on the texture and flavor of the food. What a gift is the sense of taste. Be in awe that you can chew, taste, and swallow. Wonder that you are able to feed yourself. Consider how

taste adds joy and pleasure to your day. Taste is such a marvelous thing.

5. **Touch:** Touch your loved ones—a simple gesture of hello or good-bye. Such a simple, everyday activity. Notice the texture of their skin. Feel the warmth of their skin. Touch is astounding! What would life be without touch? You can feel. Look at your hands. Gaze at your fingers. Move them. Consider what gifts touch brings to you—professionally and personally.

CHAPTER 3

Keep Tragedy in Perspective

PATIENTS ARE IN a dependent position. They are the care receiver: you are the care provider. They are guests in your "house" (the hospital) and take their cues from you. It is crucial that all members of the health care team demonstrate, even embody, hospitality as they welcome patients into their house. (After all, both *hospital* and *hospitality* are terms that share the same root as *hospitable*.)

The goal of the healer-patient relationship is to attain the patient's investment in and commitment to his or her health. With this self-investment, the patient becomes cooperative in the plan of care you and the patient cocreate. Patients are seen in a more positive light when they are understood to be cooperating in their health care, rather than complying with your plan of care. The stronger the rapport between you and your patient, the greater the patient's cooperation in his or her care will be.

The relationship with your patients is a key element in the care you provide and in your patient's experience of that care. Instill in your heart and soul the awareness that your individual self is an important, if not vital, element in the care you offer patients. You as a person matter deeply to your patients, and the way your patients perceive and experience you affects patient outcomes. Here is an experience that highlights the healing power of your person.

KATHY'S STORY: HEART TO HEART

Kathy was an active young adult until her unexpected spinal cord injury rendered her a quadriplegic. Her husband, parents, siblings, and friends surrounded her with love and support. Early on, it was clear that her life was not in danger. The health care team performed diagnostics to determine the extent of the injury and to weigh the options and prospects for treating her.

The doctor convened a meeting with Kathy and her husband, parents, and other family to review the test results. The nurse and chaplain were also present. Those results would provide a fairly reliable picture of Kathy's options. The patient possessed capacity and was able to communicate with nods of her head as well as with limited speech, which her family understood.

The doctor began by describing what the diagnostics had revealed. He then went on to describe the options and the accompanying possible risks and benefits. "Unfortunately," he stated, "the medical care you need is only available in other states. You will need to leave Albuquerque." The room was somber. Now the patient and her loved ones understood the severity of her situation. In addition, they had a grasp of the reality of her injury. The room grew silent.

After a moment, the physician began to talk personally about his family. He was a husband and father. He and his wife had children. He spoke empathetically and compassionately. He addressed the patient, acknowledging her thoughts and feelings. He looked at the family, saying that as a father, he could only imagine what was going through their hearts and minds. He said, "I wish there was more I could do." His voice cracked. There were tears in his eyes.

Kathy smiled at the doctor. He had shown her compassion and provided her hope that she could find the medical care that offered her some possibility of improvement. Likewise, her husband and her parents also thanked the doctor for the care he had provided and for giving them hope that "something could be done."

As the doctor left the room, he heard several thank-yous. He thanked them in turn. He said he would be in the unit for a while and would welcome any questions that came to mind. Saying good-bye, he left the room.

This physician was honest, authentic, caring, and self-revealing. His honesty was present in his appraisal of his ability, and that of the hospital, to offer further help to this patient. What Kathy needed was another setting that could provide the level of care that would benefit her. He empathetically discussed the seriousness of her situation and its impact on Kathy and her family. He went on to identify himself as more than a physician when he discussed his role as a parent. In doing so, he was being self-revealing.

He continued in this personal disclosure by communicating his sensitivity to the feelings of the patient and family. His tears signaled how he was touched by the challenges facing the patient and by his own pain, and he expressed his hopes for the patient as she continued to seek improvement. By sharing both his clinical insights and personal disclosures, he was able to help the patient and family begin to heal. The patient and family knew that this person, this healer, cared about them, demonstrated that they were important, and imparted the message that they mattered to him.

In general, healers are innately people of compassion. You are touched by the plight of patients. You want to relieve suffering. You want to restore function. Your compassion is a sacred gift, one requiring attention, nurture, and care. Without being mindful of the importance to nurture and refresh your compassion capacity, you may be susceptible to what is termed *compassion fatigue* or, what I call *caring fatigue.*

There are practices of self-care that are of benefit to your compassion capacity. One such practice is to stay in the moment. This means to focus on the particular patient in your care at that moment. Do your best to concentrate on this patient, avoiding, or at least minimizing, the temptation to think about how many more patients remain to be seen. Moving through your day one patient at a time will help preserve your compassion.

A second self-care practice is that of listening to your inner voice. Sensing that you are close to reaching your human limits of being present in the midst of pain and pathos is a signal to you from your heart and soul. That signal is to exercise some self-care: take several deep breaths, go to the break room for a cup of coffee or glass of water, gaze out the window at nature, or spend a few minutes with a trusted colleague. Your compassion may be so drained that you owe it to yourself and your patients to take a few days off from work.

BRANDON'S STORY: "HOW MUCH MORE OF THIS CAN I TAKE?"

A teenage athlete was rushed to the emergency room. Brandon and his teammates had been practicing that afternoon. After completing a section of his practice, he did not get up from the field. He did not move. He made no sound. The coaches and his teammates rushed to his aid and promptly called 911. When the ambulance arrived, paramedics whisked Brandon to the hospital. Within a short time, the emergency room waiting area was filled with coaches, school administrators, teammates, friends, and the patient's family. All of them were scared, mystified, and hopeful.

The health care team began to work quickly and expertly with the teenager. What they discovered was a heretofore latent anomaly—one that was life threatening. For some reason, on that particular day, at that particular time, this anomaly manifested itself, ending this young athlete's life. The situation was irreversible. Nothing coiuld be done to save his life.

With heavy hearts, the physicians met with Brandon's family. They explained as best as possible what had happened. They assured the family that the health care team did everything within its powers to help their son. They offered their sympathies and condolences to the family. After viewing their son's body, the family left the hospital in shock and sorrow. That shock and sorrow affected those who had gathered at the emergency room and the health care team as well.

The healers in the procedure room with that patient experienced an enormous drain on their compassion. Wanting so desperately to help this youth, they realized that his situation was out of their hands. When they delivered the sad news to the family, their hearts were touched as they witnessed and experienced the family's grief and hurt. Standing there with their own pain and sorrow, now they were involved in the family's pain, empathetically saddened for them. No one was left unmoved by the tragedy of that day.

Healers are dedicated to helping. When situations present themselves and it is clear that a patient is beyond the reach of what medicine has to offer, healers may feel helpless. In this episode, the healers were hit with two painful blows: the patient was a teenager and they were powerless in light of his condition. Added to their personal sorrow was their sorrow for the family. This family lost a child. The tears, groans, and grief-stricken faces all deeply affected the healers.

To a greater or lesser degree, members of the health care team who responded to this patient wondered, "How much of this can I take?" It is a violation of a universal principle when the young die: infants, children, adolescents are not supposed to die. Teenagers are full of life—active and healthy with a bright future ahead. Parents are not supposed to bury their children.

When you ask yourself, "How much of this can I take?" it is a signal to you that your compassion capacity has experienced a significant blow. This question, perhaps in other forms, will appear time and again throughout your career—expect that to happen. There is nothing wrong with you. You are not weak or afraid. To the contrary, you are caring and compassionate. Rather than worry that this question comes to you, think about what you need in order to be comforted.

Take a moment to reflect on your sources of energy and

endurance. What resources replenish your compassion? Remember—you are resilient! You have had previous life and professional experiences that staggered you. You made it through those moments, and you will come out on the other side of this particular challenge. Be kind and gentle to yourself. Draw comfort and encouragement from those sources that soothe your soul and ease your heart—music, silence, nature, exercise, solitude, trusted friendships, prayer. You will rebound.

Prayers, Meditations, and Reflections

Numbers and Patients: Keeping My Perspective

My world is largely one of numbers. I talk in numbers. I think in numbers—amount, quantity, frequency, weight, range, ratios, dosage, degree, size, stage, volume, mass, values, intake, output, time. Numbers are my gift—and my challenge. Patients depend on me and my gift of numbers.

Patients are not numbers. Numbers are in the service of people, actual persons who are husbands, wives, siblings, children, individuals. Help me to keep my patients foremost. My patients have names, loved ones, dreams, fears, quirks, admirable qualities, a past, yearnings, and future hopes. Each patient fills me with passion to do my best to bring them hope and healing. Remind me that my ability with numbers is in itself fueled by this passion. Amen.

Medicinal Powers

I thought it was my prescriptions, interventions, and treatments that helped my patients improve. That perception is certainly true. However, I have learned that there is more to the picture. My discovery is how important I, personally, am to my patients' well-being.

My compassion, my interest, and my presence with my patients all make significant contributions to how well my patients do. They trust me. They sense that I am committed. Their confidence in me magnifies the benefit of my interventions. My care for them lowers their anxiety. My presence puts them at ease—mentally, emotionally, physically, spiritually. Being calmer, their minds and bodies are more tranquil as seen in reduced worry; lowered respiration rate, pulse rate, and metabolic rate; and lessened muscle tension. When I meet with my patients, help me recall that my interactions are as important as my interventions. Amen.

Commitment Is a Process, Not an Event

How much longer can I put up with this pressure-packed, regulation-ridden, ever erratic world of health care? Policies and procedures are initiated today and expected to be followed, only to be altered or dropped tomorrow. Targets and goals continue to elevate, with quantity appearing to count more than quality—even with all the talk about patient safety and excellent care.

All I want to do is care for my patients and to have pride and fulfillment in my efforts. Some days I simply want out or find it hard to force myself out of bed to get to the office, clinic, or hospital.

In such times, it is all the more important that I sharpen my focus. What is my commitment? My commitment is to being a healer. This commitment is renewed day-by-day, sometimes hour-by-hour. It keeps me here, even in the midst of all the frustration. My commitment affects me, as well those who turn to me for help. When my commitment slips and sags, be my rod and staff, upholding and supporting me.

May I be wise enough to find another path in life if my commitment evaporates. May I be persistent and dogged enough to stay the course in what matters so much to me. Amen.

CHAPTER 4

See the Patient as a Person

WHEN TREATING a patient, it is of utmost importance to place emphasis on the *person*, not the diagnosis. First and foremost, healers engage a person—a person who seeks help. This person certainly has an illness or an injury, but the foreground in this picture of healing is the person and the background is the diagnosis. People have health problems. Health problems do not exist independently of the person. The first act of healing is to acknowledge the personhood of the patient.

A patient is a person with a rich and broad life history. The time you spend seeing a patient in your office, an exam room, a hospital floor or unit, or a treatment area is akin to viewing one scene of a feature-length movie being filmed on location. People are amazing, and your patients bestow a sacred privilege to you when they reveal their hearts and souls. You are granted immediate intimacy as they discuss and reveal aspects of their lives that are known to only a few confidants—if known at all by others. They guide you through a tour of their lives, a tour on which they reveal their disappointments, joys, achievements, hurts, trials, and triumphs.

Actually, in the span of three to five minutes, your patient will reveal deep secrets, joys, fears, and regrets, all of which have added contours and shades to this person's life. Engage the patient as a caring and compassionate guest, one who is eager, curious, and respectful. No doubt you have experienced those patients who actually inspire you and remind you why you became a healer in the first place.

Viewing someone as merely "one more patient" in the list of that day's patients will blind your eyes, deafen your ears, and close the door to your soul. You will deprive yourself of the rich vistas and stirring symphonies awaiting you upon the conversation with the patient (person) before you. Additionally, the more you come to know the person that is your patient, the more likely your treatment will be effective, as that treatment is fashioned by your acquaintance with this person and your experience with his or her injury or disease. You will have a better knowledge of what will help this person and of how this patient will tolerate and respond to the treatment you are considering and will recommend.

In the course of providing care, you are compassionate, but you are also dispassionate. The care you provide is nonpreferential. Compassion moves you to relieve or resolve the patient's health problem. Being dispassionate permits you to focus on how best to treat the patient. Providing treatment and care, you have developed the ability to compartmentalize your thoughts and feelings. You are able to focus first and foremost on what you need to do. The emphasis is more on your actions, less on your feelings, and more on your thoughts, less on your emotions. Restated, you are able to put the patient first while you fade into the background. This shift in consciousness becomes second nature to you. It requires no effort, no thought. It becomes as natural as breathing—unnoticed, yet vital to your role.

Some patients are eager to engage with a doctor and focus on their health. Others can be much more reticent, or even uncooperative. Prisoners from the criminal justice system present special and demanding problems. The primary challenge is safety—the safety of the staff and the safety of the other patients on the floor. When prisoners are on the floor, certain policies are in place and unique protocols are observed. Prisoners who are patients have a guard in their room and are generally shackled to their bed. Some prisoners can be pleasant and cooperative while others are belligerent and aggressive. Here is an episode that portrays a health care team's challenge to stay focused on the patient's health care needs rather than his status as a prisoner.

Raymond's Story: Enter This Room at Your Own Risk

Raymond was brought to the hospital in handcuffs, escorted by two guards. Once in his room, he was handcuffed to his bed. Members of the nursing staff were aware of his status as a prisoner and were observing proper procedures as they interacted with him. The nurses felt protected with the guard outside the door and with Raymond handcuffed to his bed. With their safety secured, the nurses and other members of the health care team were able to concentrate on Raymond's health care needs.

The next day, Raymond asked his guard to unlock his handcuffs so that he could go to the restroom. Once Raymond was freed from the handcuffs, he began to fight with the unarmed guard. In that struggle, Raymond grabbed an IV pole that was in his room and wielded it as a weapon. He ran to the window and attempted to smash it. After several unsuccessful blows to that window, he turned and attempted to force his way into the hall.

Once again, he and the guard began wrestling halfway in the

room and halfway in the hall. A visitor on the floor, hearing the commotion, stepped into the hall. Sizing up the situation, he grabbed Raymond from behind in a bear hug.

As soon as Raymond began his attack, the nurses called 911 and the hospital's own security officers. When the members of security arrived, they quickly restrained the prisoner, who was returned to his room and handcuffed to his bed. The police arrived quickly and began to interview the guard as well as the staff. Visitors and the staff alike were caught up in the struggle of the patient and the guard, the intervention by a visitor, the arrival of the hospital's security, and the presence of the police. The prisoner's attack created an environment of fear for those charged with his care.

The nurse directors and managers convened the nursing staff to check on the staff's physical and emotional well-being. One or two of the nurses had bruised arms. All of the nurses were upset. The hospital critical incident support team was on hand and worked with the involved nurses.

Members of the staff who were affected by the scuffle were asked if they wanted to complete their shift or if they wanted to go home. The next question was: "Who is willing to take care of this patient?" The critical incident support team assured the staff that each nurse's decision would be respected.

Violence is no stranger to hospitals. Visitors, members of the local community, disgruntled employees, angry ex-spouses (or current spouses), and team members are capable of acts of violence in hospitals. Patients can be belligerent and aggressive, subjecting the staff to spitting, hitting, or grabbing. In Raymond's story, it is a prisoner who is the violent patient.

No matter what Raymond had done to be put in prison, the staff now knew he was a dangerous person. His social status as a prisoner—and now his identification as a "dangerous person"—held the potential for obscuring his third status as a patient. As a consequence of his behavior, the hospital instituted stricter safeguards to ensure the staff's safety and to prevent another attack from Raymond. Once a safe environment was created, the question remained of whom among the nursing staff would be willing to take him as their patient during their shift.

The nurses asked this question knew their decisions would be honored. Yes, there were those who chose not to have Raymond as one of their patients. Others volunteered to take him during their shift. Their willingness demonstrated courage, compassion, and a commitment to ensure that he received appropriate care. Fear, and possibly prejudice, became secondary to other considerations.

Sometimes it is not a patient's standing in society that obscures the person behind that stereotype. On occasion, a patient's treatment decisions challenge your ability to stand by that patient. Patients frequently draw upon their religious or spiritual traditions to shape their care. The Jehovah's Witness patient refuses to be transfused with whole blood, a refusal rooted in the patient's faith community and his or her commitment to that faith. Given the widespread availability of substitute blood products, this issue in patient care has greatly diminished. Nonetheless, there are those moments when only whole blood will suffice. What follows is a story of a patient's wishes that were reluctantly honored by the health care team.

LIZ'S STORY: NO TRANSFUSIONS!

Liz was a critically ill patient whose status was being constantly monitored. She knew, as did her family, that she might require emergency surgery in order to save her life. Preparing for this possibility, the health care team spoke with Liz about her treatment preferences.

Liz understood the precariousness of her situation and grasped the jeopardy to her health. She signed the consent forms for the surgery, if it was required. She would not sign the consent for whole blood transfusions, however. She was quite clear about her reasons for that decision—her faith as a Jehovah's Witness. Liz's health care team and her family assured Liz that her preferences would be honored.

Not long after the conversation, Liz's vital signs plummeted. Every second counted. Doctors rushed her into surgery. During the procedure, Liz began to hemorrhage. The team members in the operating room did their best to stop the bleeding, but their efforts were unsuccessful. Given Liz's explicit instructions that she was not to receive a transfusion, what the operating room team would have done in similar situations was not an option. They knew what was about to unfold. Within the constraints of Liz's treatment preferences, they did what they could to stop the bleeding. Sadly, it became clear that Liz was beyond their reach.

Liz's case was heart wrenching for the entire team. The staff on her floor, the surgical team, and her primary care physician knew Liz. Her death was a blow. In the mind of the health care team, "all she needed" was a transfusion. Those who had taken oaths to do no harm and who were dedicated to patient well-being were simultaneously bound to honor Liz's preferences.

What the health care team "wanted"—or the routine clinical procedures required in a similar instance to save a life—was put aside to observe her wishes.

The impact of Liz's case on members of the health care team persisted for quite a long time. In the days and weeks following her death, members of the team met one another in the hospital and would ask, "How are you doing?" Given their commitment to honoring Liz's preferences, they silenced their own personal and professional instincts, doing so with great sorrow.

PRAYERS, MEDITATIONS, AND REFLECTIONS

Angels in Disguise

Am I not the helper? After all, I have the credentials, the education, the competencies, all of which qualify me to offer help to people with health problems. What I now realize is that there are those patients who help me! There is really no way to predict which of my patients will brighten my day. It may a young or old patient, a sophisticated or simple patient, an international or culturally different patient, a recognized or unknown patient—there's no way to tell.

What I do know is that they—unknowingly—lift my spirits, deepen my awareness, move my heart, and reignite my vision of why I am a healer. Thank you, Holy One, for these angels in disguise who brighten my day. Amen.

Behind Every Diagnosis, There Is a Person

Without a clear diagnosis, there cannot be a plan of care or a treatment regimen. It is required of me as a healer that I assess and diagnose the patient. It is my professional duty and obligation to do so. May my heart, hand, and mind be finely tuned and honed for this obligation as I serve patients.

At the same time, patients are people, not diagnoses. In my world, it so easy to refer to people as "the diabetic in Room 143," rather than "Miss Jones in Room 143 who I am seeing today for her diabetes." No one enjoys being identified or described one dimensionally, such as "the person with the green eyes," "the brunette," "the tall person," "the short person," "the knee replacement," "the preemie." People are multidimensional, so much so that they defy encapsulation. People are dynamic, unfolding, mysteries of depth and richness. Help me to maintain my wonder and respect for the people who entrust me with their well-being. Amen.

In the Presence of the Divine

READING

O LORD, our Sovereign,
how majestic is your name in all the earth!

You have set your glory above the heavens.
Out of the mouths of babes and infants
you have founded a bulwark because of your foes,
to silence the enemy and the avenger.

When I look at your heavens, the work of your fingers,
the moon and the stars that you have established;

what are human beings that you are mindful of them,
mortals that you care for them?

Yet you have made them a little lower than God,
and crowned them with glory and honor.
You have given them dominion over the works of your
   hands;
you have put all things under their feet,
all sheep and oxen,
and also the beasts of the field,
the birds of the air, and the fish of the sea,
whatever passes along the paths of the seas.

O LORD, our Sovereign,
how majestic is your name in all the earth!

—From Psalm 8 of the New Revised Standard Version
Bible (Oxford University Press, 1991)

PRAYER

In the presence and face of each patient, I behold the Eternal, the Divine. May I be humble and in awe of the divine embodied in my patient. Amen.

All Persons Are Equal in the Eyes of Health Care

We healers are just as human as anybody else. We are tempted to play favorites. We pull strings for our friends, family, and colleagues to see that they have access to the health care they need. There are those patients and families to whom we are attracted, and there are those patients and families whom we would rather avoid.

Be that as it may, when we enter a room, somehow we focus on the needs of this particular patient—regardless of his or her demeanor, social status, economic level, or educational accomplishments. All those societal standards evaporate, permitting us to see an actual person who needs our help.

Keeping Focused on the Main Thing

I have helped a lot of patients who were not nice people—violent, abusive, corrupt, manipulative, self-serving, thoughtless individuals. Aware of who they were, and what they had done, I took care of them. They were my patients. I figure that the only way I can do this is because I know who I am—a healer—which is more important than who they are in the eyes of society. Regardless of their standing, when I see them, I am the healer and they are my patients. That is the main thing.

Staying Connected

I do my best to give my patients good advice. I have a lot of experience and a wealth of knowledge. Most of the time my patients see the wisdom in my suggestions and adhere to the plan of care I outline for them. Often, there are those patients who follow a path I would not advise. They may refuse a treatment or procedure that would be of benefit, or they may embark on a path of care that offers little or no benefit while exacting a toll on themselves and their families. Help me, Source of Care, to stand by those patients who make decisions not in keeping with my professional recommendation and personal values. I do not walk in their shoes. I do not see the world through their eyes. It is not my life that bears the consequences of their choices. They still trust me and count on me. They want to know that I stand by them, honoring the path they have selected. Grant me the compassion to be supportive and attentive as I accompany them on their path. Amen.

CHAPTER 5

Practice Self-Care

PATIENT INTERACTIONS require a lot of energy. You grow so accustomed to the pace and intensity of your day that you tend to minimize the energy—physical, mental, emotional, spiritual—that you are expending in your patient interactions. Every so often, it is important to step back and catch your breath. While people can be intriguing, they also can be exasperating! They may be pleasant or perplexing. After attending to a difficult patient—one who was antagonistic or disagreeable—you long to put that interaction behind you. After all, you are reluctant to add the weight of that moment to the multiple responsibilities and worries you already carry. Nonetheless, it nags at you, in spite of your self-instructions to "forget about it" and "put it behind you." The persistence of your feelings about that patient may be a surprise to you.

You are, after all, a human with a soul, a body, and a mind. Yes, you, too, are a person first and a professional second. Many moments of your day are intense. Whether or not you experience intense feelings and emotions is not the question. Rather, the question is, "How will you manage your feelings and emotions in such a way that they contribute to your well-being?"

"Personal time" is a luxury rarely present in your day. There are always patients to be seen, cases to be treated, meetings to attend, and documentation to be completed. It is not unusual for you to ignore the demands of your body for food, sleep, or bathroom breaks. Where on earth will you find time for self-care?

Time is a reality, but it is not a barrier to self-care. It is possible to practice self-care briefly and effectively. For example, deep breaths are cleansing and relaxing. Draw in a deep breath, one that pushes against your belt. Breathe in deeply and slowly. Release that breath gently. One such deep breath can help you relax and center yourself. See if you can take four such measured and deliberate deep breaths. If not four breaths, then one breath is better than none. You are going to take a breath anyway: use it to your advantage.

Or, as you move from one patient to another, use self-talk to calm or encourage yourself. Since you are talking to yourself already about previous events and anticipating the next situation, transform that self-talk into words and thoughts that have a positive impact on you. You may have a favorite phrase or saying that you already use to put things in perspective or to encourage yourself. Call that phrase to mind, and let it free you from any lingering residue from the previous moment.

Washing your hands before and after entering a patient's room is routine and required. For twenty seconds you are alone, standing at the lavatory. Rather than silently singing "Happy Birthday," hum a few bars of a favorite song. Or, use the twenty seconds for self-coaching, calling to mind a helpful phrase. Since the water is flowing from the faucet, be mindful of the water's texture, temperature, and sound. These simple practices offer you the opportunity to use those twenty second segments to wash your spirit and heart as well as your hands. You are able to cleanse your heart and soul so that you enter the next patient's room with more presence and attentiveness. Hand washing then becomes a ritual both for leaving and for entering a patient's room, one that involves not only your hands, but also your inner self.

Since your day involves moving from one patient to another, use that travel time to look out a window. Glimpses of nature offer healing. As you pass a piece of art hanging on the wall of the corridor, glance at it. It may call to mind other times and other places—ones that bring a smile to your face or trigger a fond memory.

Walking along, look in the face and eyes of those coming from the other direction. You may cross paths with a friend, colleague, or visitor. Who knows, they may say hello or smile at you. These brief exchanges of greeting and acknowledgement have the ability to lift your spirits.

Through the course of your day, there are moments when you are alone—documenting at a desk, sitting at a computer, or making a phone call. During that time, you have a moment of solitude where you may relax and let go so that you can move on to the next patient.

Even if you are not physically alone, you may be able to slip into an internal solitude, one found within the interior of your heart and mind. Time permitting, you may turn to one or two trusted colleagues in the hall, at the nurses' station, or in the break room. It only takes a few words and a few minutes to confide in these colleagues, who extend understanding and encouragement to you. For example, even the brief quip, "Is it Friday yet?" communicates to others that your day is challenging. It is also a utilization of humor, which in itself is healing. There is no need for you to elaborate on this quip or go into detail. Others get what you mean and will no doubt smile at you while echoing back the same sentiment.

Occasionally, healers turn to chaplains. Your organization may employ full-time professional chaplains. To become a professional chaplain, one must seek specialized training and education beyond the completion of divinity school or seminary. The person who successfully fulfills these requirements is eligible to become a board certified chaplain. These professional chaplains are clearly part of the interdisciplinary team, known and trusted by the staff, and available 24-7 through an on-call schedule.

With these trusted and respected members of the health care team, you know that you can be open. Professional chaplains hold confidences. They listen empathetically to your thoughts and feelings. You are able to unload your concern, frustration, exasperation, and worry. Such conversations may last a mere thirty seconds. They may contain few words, consisting more of shrugs, facial expressions, or even meaningful silence. You might just need to share a simple phrase such as, "You wouldn't believe what *they* want us to do now!" or, "If *they* come up with one more process improvement, I am going to drop my handheld device into the commode!" The length of time or amount of words does not measure the power of the conversation; rather, its depth is what matters.

What follows is the clinical episode of a well-meaning, but exasperating, mother. In her efforts to see that her son received the care she thought important, she not only frustrated and annoyed many members of the health care team, but she also actually put her son at risk.

CARL'S STORY: MOTHER KNOWS BEST

From birth, Carl's health had been fragile. He was born with multiple life-limiting and life-threatening conditions. His mother was heavily involved in Carl's care, a tireless advocate on his behalf. The professionals at multiple social service agencies, the public school, and the health care system were all involved with Carl.

Every so often, Carl required hospitalization. Most of these hospitalizations involved a critical care setting. Due to these hospital visits, Carl and his mother were well-known to the health care team. On one particular hospital stay, staff admitted Carl with aspiration-acquired pneumonia. The health care team placed him on a ventilator to elevate his oxygen level and to ease the strain on his body and also administered antibiotics.

Members of the health care team were in and out of Carl's room, monitoring and adjusting the ventilator and changing out the IV bag containing the antibiotics. Carl's mother subjected each person who came into his room to criticism. For example, she complained about trouble with Carl's bed, the TV, the room's temperature, or the time it took for someone to respond when she turned on the call light. She criticized the care of the nurses, respiratory therapists, and the doctor. Various members of the team began to refuse to take care of Carl due to the unrelenting barrage of his mother's criticisms and demands.

One day, a nurse walked into Carl's room and found his mother giving him something by mouth. The nurse voiced his concern to Carl's mother, as Carl was on strict orders not to receive anything by mouth. Carl's mother replied sharply that she knew how to take care of Carl, and what she was putting in his mouth was going to help cure the pneumonia.

The nurse was concerned about Carl's safety, as he had a compromised airway, and the substance his mother was giving him had the potential of an unfavorable reaction with Carl's medications. The nurse took his concerns to his supervisor, who in turn contacted the doctor. The situation was alarming.

When the doctor arrived, she and the nurse went into Carl's room to talk with his mother. The doctor calmly and clearly described the risks that Carl's mother's actions posed for her son. In reply, Carl's mother told the doctor that she had been taking care of Carl since his birth and knew what was best for him. On that note, the doctor informed her that she was requesting an ethics consult that afternoon to discuss how she was interfering with Carl's treatment to the point of putting him at risk. Saying good-bye to the mother, both the nurse and the doctor left Carl's room. The doctor went directly to a phone and called the ethics committee coordinator to schedule an ethics consult for that afternoon.

In this instance, the mother moved from being annoying and frustrating to the health care team to posing a great risk to her son. The doctor was troubled. Her mind was occupied by concerns for Carl's well-being and by her apprehensions about the ethical and legal ramifications of his mother's actions. She judged that a "near miss" had occurred. She was grateful and relieved that the nurse entered Carl's room at just the right time. The ethics consult would be a supportive and resourceful setting in which the doctor could converse with Carl's mother about the dangers of her actions.

Other taxing events come along that erode a healer's self-confidence. These incidents may involve your own judgment or performance or an excruciating patient care event. You may have encouraged and supported a colleague experiencing an event that shook him or her to the core. Perhaps you have had your own experience where your self-confidence suffered a serious blow. Where do you turn when you have self-doubts?

A Doctor's Story: The Loss and Return of Self-Confidence

The chaplain received a phone call from the director of the operating room, asking her to come down to the operating room area. When the chaplain arrived, the director told her that an anesthesiologist had removed himself from a surgical case. The anesthesiologist explained to the director that a recent case was upsetting him. With that information, the chaplain went to the office where the anesthesiologist waited.

As the anesthesiologist and chaplain talked, the doctor related a recent surgery that had taken the wind out of his sails. What he experienced in that case was greatly troubling him. The patient was a healthy male, and the case was uncomplicated. During the surgery, the patient had a heart attack and, in spite of the efforts of the operating room team, died on the table. The anesthesiologist was devastated.

The chaplain said very little. What she did was provide empathy, acknowledging and affirming the doctor's thoughts and feelings. The anesthesiologist described his sense of being helpless and how he blamed himself for not rescuing the patient. Now he was afraid that another patient would suddenly worsen, and once again he would be powerless to save the patient. Almost in a whisper he uttered, "Frankly, I have lost my confidence."

After a few minutes, the doctor expressed his appreciation to the chaplain for listening. He stated, "That helped—thanks. I feel better. I will let the director know that I am ready to be back on the operating room schedule."

There is a healing power in putting into words those thoughts and feelings that distress us, that cause us pain, doubt, or fear. Getting disturbing thoughts off our chest does in fact lift a burden from our shoulders. This conversation could have transpired between the anesthesiologist and a trusted colleague or dear friend. When you find yourself wondering, "Who can I talk to about this?" remember that many people value and respect you. Nothing you say about your thoughts or feelings to those who care about you will diminish you in their eyes. They want to encourage and support you. Avail yourself of the healing they offer you.

Prayers, Meditations, and Reflections

Self-Care: I Am in Charge of My Own Well-Being

There is a lot of talk about the importance of self-care. We in health care tend to pay insufficient attention to our own health. We are helpers. We have high standards. (Are we perfectionists?) We see ourselves as invulnerable, able to keep going without sleep, food, or a break.

These expectations and self-images make me vulnerable to using stimulants to keep going and relaxants to rest. I ignore my diet, my family and friends, my exercise, my soul, and my well-being.

I know that I blame the "system" for what it "does to me." When I am honest, I know that I am the one who pushes myself so hard. I am not indispensable. I work with teams. I have excellent colleagues. My body, mind, and spirit require and deserve rest, diversion, diversity, and relaxation. As I prescribe or recommend wellness and preventive measures for my patients, may I do the same for myself? Is it possible that I am my most important patient?

Peace of Mind

⊟ When the patient's outcome is not as successful as expected, I want to know why, both for my peace of mind and to help me when I talk with the patient and/or family. This review is ingrained in me as a professional. I do this review not to highlight my failings or incompetence, but to learn and improve. Help me to avoid the extremes of eroding my confidence or of being blinded by my pride.

"What can I learn?" offers me improvement and peace of mind, whereas "What did I do wrong?" sets me up for blame and shame. Humility is the path to listening, looking, and learning from complications and reduced outcomes. May I be secure, courageous, and confident enough to be humble. Amen.

Am I Obliged or Dedicated?

⊟ Somehow the word *obligation* seems inadequate to describe my interactions with patients and families. I acknowledge and honor the multiple external obligations upon me as a healer, while carrying within me a deep commitment to do my best to help patients.

I am more than obligated to my patients. As a healer, I see myself as dedicated to my patients. My dedication is to their well-being. I become the servant of each patient, accommodating and caring as best I can. I know no other way—thankfully. Dedication nourishes my heart and soul in a way simply beyond the power of obligation. Amen.

Five Self-Care Practices

- ▸ Rest: Do your best to get a good night's sleep.
- ▸ Nutrition: Eat well and wisely; minimize grazing.
- ▸ Move: Be active, engage in activities of motion and exertion.
- ▸ Deep breaths: Inhale and exhale four slow, deep, and belt-pushing breaths.
- ▸ Kind mantras: Use your inner voice to speak words of assurance, confidence, and affirmation to yourself.

Five Minutes to Settle Yourself

1. Find a quiet and private setting (check your pulse to establish a benchmark).
2. Set your timer for five minutes, and assume a comfortable posture.
3. Begin to breathe deliberately—slow, deep breaths.
4. Close your eyes, select a mental picture of a soothing scene, and immerse yourself in that scene.
5. Continue your deep breathing—enjoy the scene.
6. When your timer signals the end of five minutes, gently exit that scene, and reenter the present. (Recheck your pulse. Is it lower?)

Stress Release Technique

 1. Go to one of your preferred private locations.

2. Sit comfortably (or lie on the floor or a couch if possible).

3. Breathe deeply and slowly. Imagine inhaling "relaxation" and exhaling "stress."

4. Starting with your toes, relax and release your muscle groups (begin with your toes, then progress to your feet, calves, thighs, buttocks, abdomen, chest, fingers, forearms, biceps, shoulders, face, and scalp). Continue your deep breathing.

5. As you move through your muscle groups, let your body become heavier and heavier, relaxing and sinking into the chair (or floor or couch if you are supine).

6. When it is time for you to resume your day, slowly arise from the chair (or floor or couch).

CHAPTER 6

Make Peace with the Tragic

QUESTIONS ARE PART of a healer's day. There are five questions that occur within health care. Central to patient care are the questions that arise as the healer and the patient ponder what steps best align with the medical indications at hand and the preferences of the patients. These questions are *treatment* questions. Healers pose their own questions regarding their decisions and actions. These questions are *self-review* questions. At times, other people raise questions about the healer's actions and performance, which are *evaluative* questions. Healers raise questions of "What is good?" or "What is best?" These questions are *ethical* questions. Finally, there is that question that strives to make sense from what appears senseless. This quest for sense is a question of *meaning*. I want to give attention to the last two questions: the question of meaning and the question of ethics.

Every day you see the unexplainable. Life does not always make sense. Why do the trim and fit develop heart problems? Why did that adult physically abuse that innocent infant? Why did that patient develop Alzheimer's disease at such a young age? Why do natural events create havoc on humans and nature itself—volcanic eruptions that sear and scorch terrain and forests and tsunamis that erase and redraw shorelines, devastating villages and cities? Why do humans unleash destruction on nature and other humans—oil and chemical spills pollute and poison oceans, rivers, and soil; school shootings end the lives of innocent children; theatre shootings take the lives of unsuspecting movie viewers; strip mining eats mountains and devours forests; car bombs in marketplaces kill shoppers; suicide bombers murder people gathered at houses of worship? These instances and others simply make no sense and prompt questions of meaning.

"Why" certainly is a question that seeks to make sense out of chaos. It is also a question in search of the good. Now we arrive at the ethical dimension of why. The ethical feature of why wants to know, "What good was served or benefit accomplished?" What you are asking is about justice, fairness, good and evil, right and wrong. "How could a couple who tried so hard to have a baby lose this pregnancy?" "Why was the drunk driver left without a scratch and the passengers killed in the car he or she struck while driving on the wrong side of the freeway?"

You witness violations of the rules of the universe: "Children do not die before their parents," "innocent people are not injured or killed," "a young parent does not develop a terminal disease, dying so that a spouse and the children are left without a husband and a father." From deep within you comes the cry, "It's just not fair—it is not right!"

How then do you balance the scales of justice in a world where what is "right" frequently is not present, and where what is "wrong" happens more often than you would want? Here is an illustration of a time when the right was overshadowed by the wrong.

Diana's Story: It's Just Not Right

Not everything that affects the health care team occurs inside the walls of the hospital. Patients often have to be transported to the hospital in order to receive medical attention. Generally, ground transportation serves the purpose of getting patients to the emergency department. In some health care emergencies, the patient's condition and distance from health care services require air transportation to a major health care center so the patient can receive the appropriate level of care. These modes of transportation are better known as "life flight."

One night a call came to the life flight headquarters, requesting that a helicopter be dispatched to pick up and transport Diana. The crew took off and reached their destination, where they placed the patient on the helicopter and prepared for transport. The takeoff went smoothly. Everything was going as planned.

Soon the helicopter was speeding through the night sky to the hospital. The crew was in radio contact with the hospital's emergency room, coordinating Diana's care with the assistance of the health care team. Without warning, the helicopter lost power and began to plummet out of control to the ground. The crash killed everyone on board—pilot, nurses, and patient. The tragic news spread like a wildfire to the entire life flight team back at the base as well as to the community's first responders, the staff waiting at the hospital, and the general public itself.

Why did this crash happen? There was nothing unusual about the flight. The life flight team was responding to a patient in need. The patient depended on the team to get her to the care she required. The staff at the destination emergency department was on standby to receive this patient and rush her to the operating room, where the surgical team was on alert. Colleagues and friends of the life flight crew were devastated. The patient's family and friends were in shock. This accident made no sense. It was wrong!

This compelling and tragic story illustrates on a large scale what happens frequently in the world of health care. Beyond the clinical features of a situation that help you understand what happened to a particular patient, there remain larger whys—the why of meaning and the ethical why. How healers respond to these crises varies from person to person. There is no blueprint or correct answer to such tragedies. Remaining in health care requires that members of the interdisciplinary team find a path that helps them move through these events. Some will turn to religion. Some will turn to a philosophic view. Whatever the chosen or preferred approach taken, the outcome needs to be one that helps you put such events in perspective so that you can persevere and continue in your vital role of serving others.

Anger, cynicism, and despair are energy depleting and passion dampening. These attitudes cannot sustain you, and they are able to affect negatively your physical, emotional, mental, and spiritual well-being. Preferably, you will fashion your own approach to tragic or senseless events, an approach that brings peace to your intellect, heart, and soul. Crafting this outlook is as essential as acquiring the skills and knowledge needed to be a healer.

There comes a time when the question of why pays you a personal visit. You may have had your own near misses with your patient, those times when you caught a miscalculation or were able to stop and contain an unexpected and unwelcome patient care event. Such moments are signaled by the "phew" that issues from you.

At other times, things happen to your patient—things beyond your control. Here is a patient care moment that depicts the widespread and devastating impact of a tragedy—an impact striking the patient, her family, and the broader health care team.

BRENDA'S STORY:
SORROW BEYOND EXPRESSION

Brenda and her husband were thrilled with her pregnancy. After two previous attempts at conceiving that ended in lost pregnancies, this pregnancy was going quite well. Brenda was in her third trimester! The grandparents were thrilled, and the health care team was happy. The nursery was ready, and her delivery date was on the horizon.

One morning, Brenda woke up as usual and began her day. Soon, she realized that she could not feel her baby moving. She waited a few minutes, trying to calm herself by thinking that her baby would move at any minute. She rubbed her stomach and talked to her baby. No movement. She alerted her husband and immediately phoned the doctor. The doctor told her to go straight to the hospital, where she would be admitted to the labor and delivery floor.

Following that phone call, Brenda and her husband headed to the hospital and were taken to their room. They had called the grandparents, who soon arrived. Brenda was scared and crying. It was unusual for her baby not to move. "What was wrong?" raced through her head. Her husband, too, was frightened, and he did all he could to comfort and reassure his wife.

Quickly, the attending obstetrician appeared at Brenda's bedside. The doctor introduced herself and said that she wanted to see what was going on with Brenda's baby. An ultrasound machine was in the room, and after prepping Brenda, the physician looked at the image on the screen. Brenda and her husband were watching as well. On the screen was their baby—motionless. There was no sound of a heartbeat. Brenda stared at the screen in silent shock. A hush came over the entire room.

Silence gave way to sobs as waves of sorrow washed over everyone. Brenda's husband held her as they both cried. The grandparents hugged one another. The sonogram technician silently shut down the machine and rolled it back to the corner. The physician took Brenda's hand and said with tears in her eyes, "I am so sorry for you and your family. Let me know if I can do anything you. I will be back in a bit, and we can talk about next steps." (The discussion of the pending induced labor and delivery awaiting Brenda could wait while she and her family reeled with their shock and grief.)

"Why?" was searing through the hearts and minds of Brenda, her husband, and their families. She had come so far in this pregnancy, and now to lose her child in utero? Her husband was crushed, simply limp with grief. The grandparents were sad for their children who had been through so much in trying to have a family.

Out in the hall, word quickly spread among the health care team. All those gathered at the nurses' station—nurses, other doctors, the chaplain—were crestfallen. The obstetrician was sorrowful for the baby, the mom, and the gathered family. This ever-expanding circle of sadness gathered up many in its arms.

One of the labor and delivery nurses was particularly upset. Helen was surprised, even caught off guard, by the intensity of her feelings. She left the nurses' station and headed to the break room to regain her composure. What surprised Helen was that she was a seasoned labor and delivery nurse who had seen just about everything. Now, Helen found herself mad and sad as the question of why resounded again and again in her heart. She had to sit down to absorb what she was feeling.

Brenda's story is tragic, inflicting a pain beyond comprehension. Helen's struggle with why is no stranger to health care professionals. This particular why is not a clinical question. Helen and her colleagues know the clinical dynamics of in utero fetal demise. Her question is not a factual one; it is a meaning question. It is a question of the heart and soul.

Prayers, Meditations, and Reflections

Integrity Precedes Accountability

The web of accountability in which I move has multiple strands. I am accountable to my profession's requirements and codes of conduct. I am also accountable to the expectations and requirements of my unit, my supervisor, my organization's targets and expectations, patient satisfaction surveys, and dozens of other regulations and standards.

Statements of accountability do not make an ethical healer. My personal integrity as a healer guides my patient interactions. No one can be forced by accountabilities to provide quality care. There are ways to meet the letter of accountability without providing the best possible care.

The patients who come to me deserve the best care I can offer. When I go home at night, I am at ease in my heart and soul, not because I met accountabilities, but because I did my best. There's nothing like feeling good about the quality of care I provided to give my body, mind, and spirit some well-deserved rest.

"It's Just Not Right!"

No one prepared me for the unexpected misfortune and tragedy visited upon my professional friends and colleagues. These are good people, giving their lives to help others. Without warning, they find themselves injured or killed in a vehicular or cycling accident. They drop dead while jogging. They are diagnosed with an aggressive cancer or other terminal condition or disease. Some successfully take their own lives, while others succumb to substance addition and abuse. These are my friends, my colleagues, my acquaintances at the hospital—not my patients! My grief and pain are different from that incurred with my patients.

In these moments, teach me to request support and to receive the comfort and consolation offered to me. Grant me the humility and courage to move from being the caregiver to being the care receiver. Free me from the illusion that I am invulnerable, implacable, and unscathed by life's sorrows—my sorrows. Open my heart and soul to this paradox: "Blessed are those who mourn, for they shall be comforted."

The path to healing from my mourning leads me through the pain, not around it. Be with me as I journey through the valley of the shadow of death, and bring me to life's pools of clear water and green pastures. Uphold me with your rod and staff, steadying me as I reel from the blow life has dealt me. Amen

Say Good-bye to Should

The word *should* can be so toxic. In my better moments, the word *should* is a friendly instructor, safe-guarding me. When moments of self-doubt arrive, *should* becomes a hostile accuser, heaping blame on me either for what I "should have done" or for what I "should not have done."

Holy One, only your forgiveness can free me from the grip of *should*. I pray for forgiveness, accepting my accountability for what transpired. Being forgiven by You, I am able to forgive myself. May I be as gracious and forgiving to others as You are to me.

Forgiveness helps me to learn from the past, to reshape my behavior in the present, and to prepare for what the future will bring. Thank you for the courage and peace forgiveness brings me. Amen.

Substitute "What" for "Why"

"Why?" is a shovel that digs a bottomless pit. With every answer I make to why, the pit is only dug deeper. The whys march at me in a continuous line, with no end in sight.

"What?" is the only antidote to why. What gives me courage. When I begin to ask, "Now what?" I turn my attention from the past (which cannot be undone) to the present and the future. In light of what has happened, what will I do today? Given past circumstances, what actions will I take in the tomorrows stretching before me?

Sustaining Presence, be my caring and wise guide, keeping me on the path of what so that I live today fully and await tomorrow's arrival with open arms. Amen.

Resiliency One-a-Day Vitamins

1. Recall previous trials where you came out OK.
2. Inventory those coping skills that you call upon in times of distress.
3. Say positive things to yourself about your ability and stamina.
4. Picture yourself successfully navigating this ordeal.

CHAPTER 7

Find Balance

HEALERS AND PATIENTS routinely weigh the health care options available to improve the patient's health and well-being. What you face as a healer is a perplexing tangle of outcomes, benefits and risks, patient preferences (cultural, religious, spiritual, values), standards of care, your professional code of ethics, and your personal conscience. Sorting through this tangle engages you in questions of ethics.

At one end of the ethical continuum is that patient who declines health care options that clearly have a treatment goal and may bring the patient significant benefits. At the other end of the continuum is that patient (and family) who demands certain steps that offer no benefit, have no treatment goal, and, indeed, may well contribute to the patient's suffering. The following example concerns a man who declined an option that would save his life. While the option before him was certainly of some magnitude, it fell well within the range of routine care, as well as acceptable and widespread standards of care. Here is the case.

JASON'S STORY: WHEN BEING ABLE TO WALK MEANS MORE THAN LIFE

When Jason was admitted to the hospital, his presenting problem was a profoundly infected lower leg. He was a diabetic, and a wound had developed. He was not fond of physicians, so he did not seek medical attention as the wound worsened. Eventually, the wound festered to the point that gangrene developed. Jason's grandchildren discovered the wound due to the stench and immediately took their grandfather to be seen by a physician, who admitted the man to the hospital.

Jason was an avid and active hiker. He loved the outdoors. When his wife died some years ago, hiking was what kept him alive. Hiking gave him a purpose, a routine, and played an important part in his coping with the loss of his beloved companion.

When the health care team examined his wound, it was clear that Jason needed an amputation. The wound was too infected, and the gangrene posed a real and imminent threat to his life if the surgery was not performed. When his health care team explained his situation and the remedy for this medical problem, Jason declined the treatment. In his mind, if he lost his leg, he would no longer be able to hike. In that case, life was not worth living.

The surgeons were set back by his reply. In their minds, the amputation was straightforward, and with rehabilitation and a prosthesis, the patient would be able to resume hiking. Jason was not persuaded and stood firmly by his refusal to have the surgery.

The health care team requested an ethics committee meeting. Jason and his two grandchildren were present, along with members of the ethics committee. The attending physicians presented the diagnosis, prognosis, and benefits that the amputation offered their grandfather. They requested that the grandchildren help Jason see the wisdom of having the surgery.

When the deliberations moved to the patient's preferences, and the consideration of quality of life, the grandchildren supported their grandfather's wishes. It was his preference, based on his values, to decline the surgery. As Jason pondered life without his lower leg, he found such a condition devoid of the quality of life he found so important. His conclusion was that it was better to die than to proceed with the surgery and lose one leg.

While the healers around the table, and those attending to the patient, were baffled by Jason's choice, they respected that decision. A course of patient care was outlined and agreed upon by Jason, his grandchildren, and the health care team.

With surgery now out of the picture, and the patient's death merely a matter of time as the gangrene progressed, the health care team moved Jason to a medical floor where he could be kept comfortable and where the wound could be kept as clean as possible. In a short time, he died with his grandchildren by his side.

This particular case is one where the patient refused the recommended treatment, resulting in his death. The health care team strongly disagreed with that choice and was deeply troubled by the patient's preference. There existed a course of treatment that would benefit Jason. The team members sensed that they had their hands tied. To them, something could be done. Yet, given the patient's preferences, they stood by, watching Jason die, knowing full well that they could help. The healers were deeply affected. It violated their dedication to help others.

You as a healer see these instances and others of less drastic and dramatic consequences where patients refuse treatment that could actually improve their health. Some less dramatic examples would be for a patient to stop using tobacco, adopt a sustainable weight-loss diet, or begin exercising (something as simple as walking). It tugs at your heart and mind to hear patients refuse to take steps that are in their best interest from your vantage point. Yet, in the eyes of the patient, that option holds no interest for them.

Your struggle may well be that of dismay. How can a patient refuse a procedure that offers benefit? In the example of Jason, he would have lost his lower leg. At the same time, he could continue his life and eventually learn to walk successfully with the help of a prosthesis. You may be bewildered by, and sorrowful at, the patient's decision.

How do you come to terms with your sorrow or frustration? It is helpful in these situations to recall that the patient is first and foremost a person. In the eyes of this person, it is no longer possible to live a meaningful and purposeful life. Life has no appeal if it is to be lived with the limitations now present due to the patient's health status.

You, like the patient, are coming to terms with life's limitations. Your wellness of body, mind, and spirit requires that you develop a perspective that enables you to consent to limitations in a way that respects and honors the patient's preferences. Simultaneously, the way you respond to those inevitable limitations determines to a great degree your personal and professional well-being.

Over the years, you will be involved in patient care situations where you are saddened by, or incredulous at, the choices patients make. You will find that their choices conflict with your commitment to their well-being. How do you take care of yourself in such instances? Does music help ease your mind? Do you find exercise (walking, cycling, or fitness classes) helpful? Is it beneficial for you to be alone or to find someone who will listen to you? Maybe reading helps you in such moments. Perhaps time spent doing yoga, meditating, or praying offer your heart and mind peace. Whatever strengthens and encourages you is the point, as these and other practices or resources of support and renewal are vital to nurturing and sustaining your resilience over the years.

Now our conversation moves to the other end of the ethics continuum. In these instances, you meet a patient and his or her family who adamantly insist on a particular intervention, one that you and your colleagues know has no efficacy and offers no benefit. No goal can be achieved by further efforts to treat the problem. Indeed, you and your colleagues are concerned that the patient will be subjected to purposeless and prolonged suffering.

A dramatic and vivid example of just such a demand is the one of keeping a patient on a respirator when such action is unable to attain any treatment goal and is devoid of any benefit to the patient. All that medical science can do for the patient has been done. The patient is actually dying due to irreversible circumstances. What the respirator and medications are doing is prolonging the patient's dying. The patient's medical condition is the clinical state of multiple organ dysfunction syndrome (MODS). Consider this instance.

THOMAS'S STORY: AGONIZING DECISIONS FOR A SUFFERING PATIENT

Thomas, a middle-aged man, collapsed at home and was rushed to the local hospital. He was stabilized, and doctors made an initial diagnosis. He had suffered a major stroke. He was unconscious and unresponsive. The health care team put Thomas on a respirator and transported him to a larger medical center in a metropolitan setting. His wife accompanied him.

At the larger medical center, the health care team moved Thomas from the emergency department to the intensive care unit. After a thorough workup, the team informed his wife that there were no further treatment options. Her husband's brain was irreparably damaged. He was able to take a few breaths on his own when taken off the respirator. They suggested to her that Thomas's care be focused on comfort, as he had only a few days left.

The patient's wife and family absorbed the sad news. The wife, the patient's brother, and the children of the patient all agreed that the patient should be taken off the respirator and that his care be designed to keep him comfortable and peaceful, with his family at his side.

However, his sister, who was alienated from the patient and who lived out of state, voiced her objection. She argued that Thomas and his wife were not legally married. While they had lived together for more than thirty years, they had not married. No common law marriage statute existed in the state. Consequently, she contended that as her brother's surrogate, she was the health care decision-maker for her brother.

Thus began a protracted battle of wills and words. In the meantime, Thomas remained on the respirator while his body continued to shut down. His physical state became gruesome. The healers involved in his care sensed that the smallest efforts of patient care (turning, bathing, lip and mouth care) only caused the patient to suffer.

Every effort to have the objecting sister come to the hospital to observe her brother, talk with the family, and sit with the health care team was brushed aside. The family was tormented as they witnessed the suffering and decline of their loved one. The situation seemed to have reached an impasse, with Thomas bearing the brunt of the family's disagreement and conflict.

Finally, one of the patient's brothers went to court, asking that he be made the patient's guardian. After hearing the details of the patient's situation, including the medical condition as well as the family dispute, the judge gave the right of guardianship to the patient's brother.

Returning from the courthouse, the brother requested that Thomas be taken off the respirator, as was the original plan. Shortly after the respirator was removed, the patient died peacefully. His wife and members of his family were with him. There were tears of sorrow and relief that his ordeal had finally come to an end.

If one word were to be chosen to describe this situation it would be *agony*. The patient certainly was in physical agony. The health care team agonized as they were obligated to continue to attend to the patient in ways that went against the preferences of the patient's wife and family. The very care they were providing was a source of torment to the patient and a cause of personal and professional moral and ethical misery as they had pledged to do no harm. The situation was horrific.

When you experience such heartrending and conscience-tormenting cases, how do you tend to your heart and soul? This moment will reappear throughout your career. These cases will present you with an ethical determination of what serves the patient's best interest and what is acceptable to your professional and personal ethics. How do you prepare for, and successfully navigate, these moments? How do you nurture and heal your heart and soul during such an ordeal? How do you nurture and heal your heart and soul once the tragedy has concluded?

As a health care professional, you have voluntarily accepted the obligation and commitment to the patient's well-being. That obligation and commitment are a mix of the patient's preferences and values and the knowledge and skills that you put at the service of your patient's well-being. A tension, if not disagreement, is inevitable given the potential conflict between those two perspectives. This observation is not evaluative. The situation is neither good nor bad. Rather, the observation is about reality. It is simply descriptive. It will happen.

You know from your life experience, as well as your experience as a health care professional, that a troubled conscience has an enormous power to distress and upset you. You will toss and turn physically, emotionally, and spiritually. You will not be at rest but in a continuing state of unrest. For your well-being, it is vital to your self-care that you put in place those steps or practices that will bring you peace.

One step is to identify your own boundaries, which will help you to be centered and prepared in the future. As a situation permits, you can refer the patient to a respected colleague. You do so with the knowledge that the referral represents the provision of good patient care while at the same respects your professional and personal integrity.

Another step is to identify, and put in place, those resources that comfort and sustain you in the midst of these extenuating situations. For the ancients, it was precisely the heart that was the seat of ethical deliberation and decision. In your search for peace for your conscience (heart), who are the trusted others in whom you may confide? What resources offer you peace of mind and conscience? Does meditation help you to listen to your intuition and inner voice? Does prayer help you sense direction and support from the Divine?

Prayers, Meditations, and Reflections

"Why?"

⤒ "Why?" is a question of my mind and my soul. My mind is pretty good at sorting out the various clinical aspects that contributed to a complication or a diminished or tragic outcome.

It is my soul that faces the more difficult search. Why did this incident happen to this patient? I can't make sense of it. My heart and soul are troubled. How do I face the tragic, the unexpected, or the unwanted? My view of life is strained, if not shattered.

Help me sit with the pain and distress stirred up by why. Help me to listen. In the distress of my heart and mind, I offer this prayer:

"God, grant me the serenity
to accept the things I cannot change;
the courage to change the things I can;
And the wisdom to know the difference." Amen.
—"Serenity Prayer," Reinhold Niebuhr (1892–1971)

Patient Care Perplexities

My involvement in caring for patients involves ethical dilemmas on a daily basis, large and small. How much do I tell the patient? I am torn between being realistic about what is in store for this patient while fostering some degree of hope. How do I describe the patient's disease progression while also being compassionate and caring? What is the best way to convey to this patient, and his or her family, that the time has come to transition from treatment to comfort care?

These questions, and others, toss and turn in my heart, soul, and mind. I am committed to doing no harm and seeking what benefits the patient. Grant me a stillness and silence so I may listen and discern. My help is found in returning and rest; in quietness and trust my strength emerges. From the depths of my heart and soul will appear the assurance and insight to guide me through the tangles currently confounding me.

Source of Stillness, when the storm waves of patient care threaten to swamp my heart and soul with the waters of worry, help me hear Your calming voice say, "Peace—be still." Amen.

CHAPTER 8

Contend with Limits and Possibilities

PATIENT CARE TRAVELS along a trajectory, stretching between cure and comfort. Along this trajectory, patients and their healers arrive at the realization that care has reached a point that requires a new approach, the approach of comfort, sometimes called *palliation*.

Comfort care does not represent a defeat or an inadequacy in any way of the diagnosis itself. It does not entail a lessening of the efforts and interventions followed to help the patient. No, comfort care represents providing the appropriate (indicated) care in the appropriate setting. Such care is in accord with the patient's medical indications and with the preferences of the patient or health care decision makers. Both curative care and comfort care are manifestations of care in the broadest sense and are both reasoned and reasonable approaches.

The trajectory of patient care occurs between the parentheses of limits and possibilities. The experience of the limits of the human body and the limits of human knowledge and healing interventions can be sobering.

JANE'S STORY: A DEVASTATED MOTHER AND FATHER

Jane, an expectant mother, appeared for her routine prenatal visit. Throughout her pregnancy, everything had proceeded as expected. On this visit, during the course of her examination, her obstetrician detected some unusual features of the fetus. The doctor referred Jane to a perinatologist. Both the mother and father waited anxiously for that appointment.

After the perinatologist performed the additional tests, anomalies were discovered that were incompatible with life. As kindly as possible, the perinatologist delivered this tragic news to Jane and her husband. Upon learning the condition of their unborn baby, the parents were crushed. They held each other, weeping silently. The future they had envisioned was now drastically altered.

This stark incident of the limits experienced in health care is tragic and heartrending. Healers are committed to helping their patients by using their skills and knowledge to benefit their patients. Such instances of intractable limits are jolting and hard to bear. With few exceptions, giving birth is routine. Mothers and fathers conceive babies, which the mother carries to term. While healthy babies and healthy moms are an everyday occurrence, there are exceptions.

Creating your own way of coming to terms with the inevitable limits that you and your patients will face is essential to your longevity in health care. Accompanying the development of your personal resources to sustain and support you in the face of limits is the task of shaping how you offer support and compassion to your patients and their families who are facing the limits of medicine. Your patients will turn to you for empathy and kindness. Your response will play a significant part in how well they manage their disappointment.

Yes, limits are no stranger to you and your patients. However, in the course of patient care, unexpected possibilities appear and introduce themselves. A "what if" manifests itself. Life is wonderfully dynamic. Situations do change. These surprising possibilities hold promise where none was initially present. The gift of this possibility—this option—offers you the hope that perhaps this patient's situation and outcome may yet be improved. For the patient, the news of this possibility and its attendant promise of benefit and improvement lifts his or her spirits and generates joy and relief. Many patient care situations contain promising moments of possibilities as well as sobering moments of limits. Consider this health care experience of unseen possibilities.

ANTHONY'S STORY: MANNA FROM HEAVEN

Anthony's kidneys had been failing and finally stopped functioning. He was a thirty-something man—a husband, a father, a person pursuing his career. Anthony started dialysis while his health care team launched a search for a suitable match for a kidney donation. First, his family was tested, which did not result in a match. The health care team entered his name on the national registry for a cadaveric transplant. The waiting began.

With the passing of time and the decline in the patient's health, the quest to find a suitable donor became even more urgent. Both the health care team and Anthony waited anxiously, hoping that with each new day word would come that a kidney was available. The patient and his family, as well as the health care team, did their best to be confident and hopeful that a kidney would be found—the sooner the better!

In the community, the public was learning about nonfamily, living donor kidney donations—a novel and much-discussed alternative approach at that time. These donations required a match between donor and recipient, with the potential donor needing to complete the extensive and comprehensive organ donation screening process.

Being accepted as a living donor was no easy accomplishment, and it required that the potential donor, in addition to meeting the requirements to be designated as a match, be a highly motivated, committed, and altruistic person. It required a person willing to undergo surgery, facing all the risks involved in a surgical procedure.

Within the community, a woman in her thirties had concluded that she wanted to help someone by volunteering to be a living kidney donor. She fulfilled all the requisite steps and was accepted onto the registry as a living donor. The matching process determined that her kidney was the best match for Anthony.

When the health care team delivered news of the availability of a kidney from a living donor to Anthony and his family, they wept tears of joy. The healers were relieved and thankful on behalf of their patient.

Who was this angel of mercy? How could this possibly be? Little or no thought had been given to the possibility that a living donor would appear. Given the privacy and confidentiality of the organ donation process, neither the donor nor the recipient knew anything about the other—only that a suitable match had been found.

The health care team set a date for the transplant. Both the donor and the recipient were prepared for their surgery, with both procedures going smoothly. Both patients did well post-surgically, surrounded by their loving and comforting families. In short order, the two patients—donor and recipient—were discharged, and they returned to their lives.

Anthony was filled with the deepest gratitude for this Good Samaritan who gave him the gift of life. The donor was filled with a profound gratitude that she had been able to participate in an once-in-a-lifetime act of kindness.

Possibilities elicit humility, for these options frequently are not the making of our own hand. Rather, they appear as gifts, as in the case of the living donor. As a healer, not only are you humbled, but you are grateful at those junctures when possibilities appear out of thin air. You are grateful that this possibility appeared, uninvoked by your skill or knowledge. With its revealing, your hope and imagination may be stirred. If this possibility is present, then how may it be expanded and enlarged exponentially to make even other possibilities available—possibility building on possibility?

DEATH: THE FINAL LIMIT OR THE NEXT PHASE?

Death is part of the cycle of life. The life cycle has beginnings and endings, coming one after the other. Clearly death may be viewed as an event fixed in time, what is called the *date of death*. Viewing death more in terms of a cycle offers a perspective wherein death becomes the conclusion of life and, at the same time, the continuation of life. Undeniably, death marks the end of an individual's life. It is also the end of a generation, with all of its contributions and its shortcomings. With the passing of individuals, and of generations, the past gives way to the future, to the next generation and the influence it will have on life. From nature, we see that winter gives way to spring or that a devastating forest fire ushers in new growth. Death is both a good-bye to what was, and a hello to what is yet to be.

For you as a healer, death may be seen as the "enemy"—even as a failure. That impression is likely to be in place if you view yourself as capable of winning a wrestling match with death. Such a view is bound to lead to the perspective of seeing death as an adversary, if not an enemy, to be met in the arena and defeated.

The art and science of healing has its limits. Patients, too, are limited: they have only so much stamina, reserve, and strength. Within the circumference of the possible, what can be done is done. Sometimes, it is simply not possible to mend a certain injury or illness; there is no failure, no defeat in such circumstances. Rather, there is recognition of what is possible and what is not possible.

Certainly a family experiences sorrow, anguish, and, perhaps, anger and guilt at the moment of death and in the days following the death of a loved one. Mourning and sorrow signal the pain of their loss while at the same time are part and parcel of the healing aspect of their grief process. You as a healer may be remorseful and blame yourself for letting down the patient and the family.

Such a view that death is an enemy to defeat is bound to lead to frustration, discouragement, or anger since death is stronger that are we. Death does not stand apart from life, waiting for an opportunity to intrude into life so as to extinguish it. No, death is embedded in life itself. Death is not a force outside life, waiting to pounce and take life. Death is more than an event. Death is a process, unfolding along with life itself. In our living is our dying.

Certainly, you will do what is within your power, and within the power of medicine at the present, to return your patients to a life of vigor. Your patients have a strong will to live—a will not only of the mind but also of the spirit and body. Your interventions support and advance this will. In most instances, the combination of your efforts, along with the stamina of the patient, cooperate in returning the patient to an active and meaningful life.

At other times, a particular patient's powers of life, and your powers as a healer, are less than the powers of death. In spite of the patient's will to live and in spite of your efforts, the patient will die. You and the patient do your combined best to hold onto life. There is no failure. There is no defeat. There is instead the realization that humans are finite—as a healer, your powers (knowledge and skill) are limited, as are the patient's powers of healing and recovery. You can only do what you can do. The patient does the best she or he can do.

Death is acutely and profoundly experiential. We humans do give thought to death and devise our own philosophical or religious/spiritual perspectives and approaches to it. At some point, death moves from being a subject of thought or reflection to being an experience. That experience may be our own pending death, the death of a loved one, or a moving news story of deaths caused by violence, disease, terrorism, or nature. In your role as a healer, death is an everyday occurrence. Each of those deaths affects you to some degree.

Intellectually or spiritually, it is one thing to understand death as integral to life itself and not some unrelated power "out there" that is life's adversary. It is another thing to experience death, specifically the death of one of your patients. Your patient's death brings you sorrow and mourning. A loved one—your patient—is no longer physically present and available to you or the patient's family. It is important for you to honor your sorrow and resist avoiding or masking your grief.

Your experience with death as a healer is diverse. Death ranges from the tragic, untimely, accidental, unexpected, and sudden to the expected, anticipated, peaceful, or awaited. How you view the death of your patients—the manner and cause of the patient's death and your relationship to the patient—all contribute to the nature and magnitude of your sorrow and mourning.

Do not be surprised at the variation of your grief at the death of a patient, as there are multiple factors of death that contribute to and influence how you will grieve. There is no question that you will grieve. However, you may question whether your grieving is healthy and healing.

Be kind and gentle with yourself as you grieve. Some patient deaths will stir, if not trouble, your heart and soul more than other patient deaths. Do your best to be at peace with the variation of the deaths and the grief you experience.

It may be that over time, a patient's death becomes a humble realization of our limits as humans and as healers. For the family and other loved ones, it may be that the sorrow, anger, and guilt slowly and eventually subside, with the gradual blossoming of a growing gratitude for the time their loved one gifted and graced their lives. For you as a healer, you may sense that against terrific odds, you did your best to serve that patient—an effort of courage and compassion. What more could you ask of yourself?

Sometimes, Comfort Is the Path to Follow

Healers always provide patient care. Caring for patients is the bedrock of health care and of what you do. In general, patient care may be viewed as occurring in two forms: *treatment* and *comfort*. These two expressions of care are not distinct spheres, but are overlapping circles. Comfort involves treatment. Treatment brings comfort. These two dimensions of patient care are present as you discern what you judge to be the appropriate care for a particular patient.

This discernment involves many dimensions and considerations for you to weigh as you deliberate which path of patient care is appropriate—helpful, beneficial—for your patient. In the fluid situation of caring for your patient, the scale at one point may be tipped more toward treatment. At other times, the scale may be tipped more toward comfort. Generally, treatment seeks to alleviate a disease or injury to a greater or lesser degree. The goal of comfort care is to alleviate pain and suffering by providing rest and peace of body, mind, and soul.

Treatment and comfort are not an either-or consideration. Both are always present. One image of the unity of treatment and comfort is that of a piano. The keys of the piano provide the musician movement up and down a tremendous range, with the low notes at one end and the high notes at the other end. The piano player's fingers move deftly, combining notes from the low, mid, and high range, creating the beautiful sounds of music.

In like manner, patient care moves up and down medicine's keyboard. This medical scale has a low, mid, and high range, permitting you to combine or highlight those aspects of care that offer the most benefit to your patient. What you are doing is truly music to the ears of your patients. United as treatment and comfort are, treatment always includes an element of comfort—as in the provision of antinausea medications during chemotherapy or pain medications following a procedure. Likewise, comfort always involves a dimension of treatment of some kind, since treating pain is itself a comfort measure. These two approaches are united by the goal of medicine: to care for the patient.

Here is a situation that illustrates the trajectory of patient care traveling along the treatment-comfort continuum of care.

Ellen and Glenn's Story: From Errands to Emergency

Ellen had been grocery shopping while her husband, Glenn, exercised on their home treadmill. When she returned from shopping, she called out his name to let him know that she was home. While putting away the groceries, she could hear the treadmill. Glenn did not reply to her calls. "Well," she thought, "maybe he has on his headset." She walked into their exercise room, where she saw the unexpected and frightening: he was sprawled on the floor, and the treadmill was running! She ran to him. Kneeling beside him, she realized instantly that Glenn was not responsive. She frantically called 911. When the ambulance arrived, Glenn was transported to the hospital, where he was admitted to the critical care unit.

Ellen was bewildered. One moment, Glenn was exercising. The next minute, he was on the floor, unresponsive. While she sat by his bedside, the health care team examined him and conducted multiple tests. They managed his symptoms as the search continued for a diagnosis and treatment options. Glenn did not respond to his wife, and his breathing was dependent on a ventilator. Ellen remained hopeful that he would wake up.

When the tests were completed, the attending doctor stopped in to talk with Ellen. He told her that the diagnostics showed that her husband had a massive heart attack and had been on the floor without a heartbeat or respiration for quite some time. The amount of time when he had neither circulation nor respiration had irreversibly damaged his brain. Consequently, Glenn no longer had any brain function at all, including the ability to breathe on his own. It was time to think about next steps.

Ellen had feared that her husband might not recover. Now the doctor's words confirmed those fears. She asked, "What are those next steps?" The physician replied, "The breathing tube is of no benefit to him. While the breathing tube is unable to help your husband, there are still things we can do. We have several options for keeping him comfortable. It is time to take him off the ventilator, remove the breathing tube, and help him be as restful and peaceful as possible."

In the course of caring for Glenn and Ellen, the health care team exercised both treatment and comfort to the degree appropriate to the patient's status. The healers explored what treatment might be effective and of benefit. Once it became clear that the patient's condition would not respond to, or benefit from, treatment, the healers transitioned their care to providing comfort to the patient and support to his wife. Through the course of Glenn's care, the healers were always caring for the patient. That care took different forms in accordance with his status. The transition from treatment to comfort is far from a failure or a defeat: it is compassionate and competent patient care.

Prayers, Meditations, and Reflections

Humility Trumps Pride

⊒ Cosmic Comforter, I pride myself in what I can do to alleviate pain, to mend injuries, and to cure diseases. My power is such that now I can prevent illness. My successes give me confidence and assurance. Help me keep my pride in check, so that it does not mutate into arrogance. Arrogance shifts my focus from the needs of the patient to me— to what I think is best for the patient, to how proficient I am, to what I can do. Grant me humility so that I may be sensitive to what my patient wants and requests. If I am to be proud, may I be proud that my patients appreciate me for the humble person and competent healer I am. Amen.

Is There a Balm for a Wounded Heart?

⊒ I am surprised at how sad I am at my patient's death. Something about this death is getting to me. I am not prepared for these feelings of sorrow that come and go. I am the one who speaks to patients' families when their loved one has died. Now I wish I had someone to talk to about my own grief. Am I weak or unprofessional? I am sad and scared of my emotions. Grant me your steadying arm, your comforting shoulder, your consoling presence, Holy One. Apply your soothing salve on my sorrowful soul. Be present in the caring words and understanding glances of my family, colleagues, and friends. Amen.

Expect the Unexpected

☐ Not always, but sometimes, when I run into a wall, I happen upon a door! I have no idea how this happens, but not knowing does not keep me from being gratefully surprised! In those moments of patient care when there are more walls than doors, may I be encouraged knowing that the unexpected can be expected. I have had it happen before.

Healing Rituals for the Griever

☐ 1. Acknowledge your sorrow. Doing so honors the affection you held for the deceased and respects your own humanity as mourning the death of someone important to you. Being sad does not mean that you are weak, bad, unprofessional, or "losing it." Your sorrow means that you cared.

2. Do your best to get adequate rest and good nutrition. Be moderate in your consumption of alcohol, caffeine, and sugar.

3. Attend the person's services (memorial, funeral, wake). These services offer healing in their rites and rituals and in the gathered company who are united in grief and who are sources of support and comfort to one another.

4. Draw upon your own spiritual and religious practices and resources. Light a candle. Say prayers. Read from sacred scripture. Speak to your spiritual or religious leader or guide. Meditate. Reflect.

5. Spend time with your spouse, trusted friend, or close colleague. Turn to these loved ones and others who will listen to you without being judgmental.

CHAPTER 9

Show Compassion

COMPASSION IS an invaluable component in your relationship with your patients. At the same time, the pathos to which you are exposed on a daily basis along with the empathy you extend to your patients and families have the power to drain you emotionally and spiritually. It comes as no surprise that you find yourself tired, since compassion means "to suffer with."

Your patients are spouses, siblings, grandparents, addicts, professionals, laborers, homeless, hobbyists, plumbers, volunteers, criminals, and members of various organizations and clubs whose worlds have now been constricted by health problems and concerns. The loss of their world as they knew it (and liked) is pushed aside by this new world (one that they did not request).

When these patients seek health care, you certainly attend to their health problems. Woven into their health problems is their grief at the loss of their former selves. Whether for a brief period of time or for the remainder of his or her days, a once-healthy person is now a patient. You sense this grief, which may present itself as anger, remorse, or despair. In the patient story below, Pete reveals the impact an illness, and a successful treatment, can have on a patient's life.

Pete's Story: "I Am Not the Man I Used to Be!"

Pete had a heart attack in his office and was rushed to the hospital. He was treated quickly and effectively. He benefited from the expedited process of moving heart attack patients quickly from the emergency department to surgery ("minutes mean muscle"). Naturally, the patient and the family were relieved that his life was saved.

Pete's initial appreciation that he survived the heart attack quickly began to fade as he was informed of his heart attack's impact on his physical stamina and strength. He now was a congestive heart failure patient. This condition required fairly significant alterations and adaptations at home and work.

This robust, hard-working, and successful businessman was deflated by this unexpected news. His deflation gave way to anger and depression, as he no longer was "the man he used to be." Pete required oxygen support 24-7 and needed to limit and apportion his activities in accordance with his significantly reduced strength and stamina.

Pete had both greater and lesser success facing his new self-image. He was grateful to his health care team, yet angry and sad at the state in which he now found himself. His family was affected as well, for the husband and father who once was an active man now was a changed and different person. Not only was he quite physically limited, his mood and outlook had been altered. A once good-natured loved one, Pete was now a bitter and forlorn man.

This case illustrates how a change in a person's health status has physical, emotional, personal, family, and spiritual consequences. You are involved in similar situations. You may touched by how the patient is attempting to contend with the pain, the alterations in self-identity and self-image, the level of physical and/or mental functioning, other discomforts, and the loss of independence that accompany change in a person's health.

Patients face actual and potential readjustments that are imbedded in their health problem. It may well be that their former lives are demolished. They realize that much of their vitality, role, identity, and activity level are things of the past; they are no longer attainable. When they consider the future, what they behold are unknowns and uncertainties, and sometimes what they imagine is unappealing and unwelcome. While the specifics may remain unclear, they do know that a health episode has forever changed the path of their lives. "Now what?" is the burning question.

Your compassion unites you with this patient as he or she faces the challenges brought by each day. Your compassion also unites you with this patient as he or she ponders what the future holds and how that future may be quite different from the one he or she envisioned prior to this health problem. A health decline quite possibly may include changed and limited diet, assumption of an exercise routine, altered levels of activity and independence in daily living, dependence on prescriptions, scheduled visits to the doctor for checkups, modifications to the patient's home to accommodate medical equipment, a changed body image due to treatments or surgeries, reductions of income, and the loss of a former self-identity requiring the development of a new identity and self-image. Your patient is no longer the person you knew.

These changes are accompanied by modification of the patient's meaning structure and sense of purpose for his or her life. "What's the point?" is a frequently heard question. Your patient struggles to find new meaning and purpose for his or her life, given present circumstances. "If I can't do that, what's the point?" This question is certainly about physical and mental function. It is also a profound question about how to find and experience meaning and purpose.

The patient's family is affected by what happened to their loved one. The person they once knew is changed. Their perception of the loved one, and their interactions with him or her, are all modified in light of their loved one's altered health status. Family roles and responsibilities may require reassignment as the family network reorganizes and adapts to their loved one's condition. New caregiving roles may be required of them to support and care for their family member as well as the broader family. They stretch the hours in their days and draw on their physical reserves to be caregivers. Simultaneously, they feel the pull on their emotions and spirits as they grieve with and for their loved one.

SUFFERING: THE SIXTH VITAL SIGN

The Greek root of suffering is *pathos*. Pathos is a multidimensional term and may be translated as "passion, suffering, feeling, or disease." In some instances, passion may be understood as suffering. The word *compassion* is generally understood to mean "to suffer with" (com-passion).

Passion may also be understood as energy or zeal ("she is passionate about music"). In contrast, *apathy* (a-pathos) is the lack of energy ("he is apathetic about his job"). Chapter 10 will examine passion as energy. The remainder of this chapter considers passion from the perspective of suffering.

What is suffering? How is suffering related to pain? Pain is connected to, yet distinctive from, suffering. Pain has become the "fifth vital sign" and is assessed by means of the pain scale, where patients are asked to give a numeric measure of their pain. The popular pain scale, ranging from one to ten, is employed: one is no pain and ten is excruciating pain. Pain is a subjective experience. Some people have a higher pain threshold—or greater tolerance—for pain than others. The pain scale captures that subjective and individual, or person-to-person, variation. The term *uncomfortable* is commonly used as a synonym for hurt or painful. The pain scale is one exception to that practice. Pain is called *pain*.

Interestingly, there is not—at present—a scale for suffering. The lack of such a scale is a cause for wonder. Suffering may be called intractable pain or a pain breakthrough. Suffering is communicated by the patient, sometimes verbally but most often through winces, contortions, groans, profound restlessness, and agitation. Those around the patient—family and healers—read the signs and realize that pain has given way to suffering.

The patient's suffering is matched by your compassion to bring relief and comfort. Suffering is pointless pain. It is pain that has no healing goal, no healing benefit. It is one thing to subject oneself to pain for the purposes of improved health—such as an immunization shot or a surgical procedure. Ironically, healing often involves hurting or feeling pain to a greater or lesser degree.

Suffering is encompassing, having an impact on body, mind, and spirit. Suffering leaves no part of the person untouched. It is pervasive. No matter the location of the identified or diagnosed pain—whether the source is the mind (troubling, disturbing, or irrational thoughts), the soul (burdens, torments), or the body (traumatic injury)—the patient's entire being reels with the anguish of suffering.

Suffering is unbearable to the patient and creates a situation for which there are few to no resources available for its management, other than perhaps sedating the patient to the level of unresponsiveness. Suffering certainly pulls at the hearts of the family, friends, and healers. Observing a patient suffer is one of the most grueling moments healers experience.

Suffering induces a sense of helplessness and meaninglessness in healers. Suffering appears to be unassailable by any efforts to relieve it. At the point of suffering, the patient is not consolable or responsive to any efforts to comfort or ease his or her body, mind, or spirit. Suffering dominates and occupies the patient entirely. Unlike pain, where there is hope and good reason to expect it to be attenuated, if not subside or resolve, suffering is a static state to which there appears no remedy or end. In general, suffering is most often manifested in those patients who are in end-of-life situations.

Human hearts break in the presence of suffering. A family does not want a loved one to suffer. You do not want to see your patient suffer. Your desire is first to prevent suffering through prevention and wellness approaches and practices. While prevention and wellness serve a great purpose, disease and injury are part of the fabric of human life. When suffering occurs, you move from prevention to treatment. Your passion is to alleviate human suffering in its holistic and multidimensional manifestation—the suffering of body, mind, and spirit.

Despair is another expression of suffering. Despair appears when patients envision a future devoid of hope. The landscape before them is bleak and barren, as harsh and formidable as a New Mexico field of volcanic rock. When patients learn that there is no treatment that will improve their situation, they are subject to despair. In moments of waiting for a test result, patients may despair that the findings will signal a profound altering of their lifestyle. They may learn from their diagnostic tests that their status will only continue to decline and worsen. Initially, a patient may be morose, or despair, and understandably so.

In accordance with the patient's meaning structure—religious or philosophical—some patients will continue to despair. In some instances, the patient's despair may give way to fury or to feeling forlorn. In this state, there is an acute awareness of isolation, of being abandoned, and of facing their dilemma alone. They may well sense that they are disconnected from God, family, and friends. There is a diminished sense of community and of connection with caring and supportive others.

Other patients will travel in this valley of the shadow of despair and come to terms with their situation within the framework of their meaning structure. Basically, they "consent" to their condition (I am indebted to Dr. James Gustafson for this definition of consent). This consent is not a resignation. As a central term in health care, consent centers around all care, with a patient or a spokesperson making an "informed consent" to suggested treatments or procedures. Informed consent is a process, an ongoing dialogue and discussion, not a document that is signed, sealed, and static.

Consent is a process in which the patient weighs the available options and alternatives, considers the benefits and risks accompanying those options, examines the treatment goals promised by each alternative, and makes a decision based on that patient's values. Clearly, consent is not deflation or defeat. It is not a posture of resignation. Quite the contrary, consent is a realistic appraisal and acknowledgement of circumstances, which culminates in the patient consenting to what is attainable. There is no railing or lashing out. The patient does not withdraw or shut down. Rather, consent brings a certain resolution, if not peace.

Patients may well demonstrate resolve, determination, and even courage knowing that the future before them is one they have reviewed. It is a future for which they have prepared. Patients continue to have some say in the course of their lives. It is not uncommon to see despair diminished, or even disappear, to the degree that the patient is able to consent to his or her future.

Here is a clinical event that highlights those moments in patient care involving suffering, despair, and consent.

DAN'S STORY: A PEACEFUL ENDING

Dan was a middle-aged male whose kidneys had failed. He was placed on in-hospital daily dialysis while his health care team reviewed his situation. His family initially hoped that he would recover and be able to leave the hospital. When it became clear that his kidneys would not recover, the health care team looked into the possibility of a kidney transplant. However, it was determined that a kidney transplant was out of the question given Dan's drastically diminished and compromised health status. Dan's situation appeared dire.

No stone had been left unturned. All the benefits that treatment options could offer this patient had been considered, implemented as indicated, and were now exhausted. For all practical purposes, the patient's dying was being prolonged by the daily dialysis treatments.

The health care team asked to meet with Dan's family to discuss his care. The healers spoke compassionately of their patient's situation, reviewing what had already been attempted and gently informing the family that sadly, there were no further effective medical treatment options.

On hearing this sobering news, Dan's son, a man in his early twenties, broke into tears. He insisted that his father continue to receive dialysis in the hospital. The health care team explained compassionately that dialysis involved significant invasive and painful procedures, serving no treatment goal and being of no benefit to his father. Dan's son brushed aside their comments. The health care team assured the son that nothing was going to happen immediately and that the dialysis would continue for a few more days. During this time, the family and healers would meet again to discuss the patient's condition.

Given the impasse, the health care team requested an ethics consult. Present at the ethics consult were members of the ethics committee, the treating clinicians, the son, and his significant other. After introductions and a description of the purpose of the ethics consult, a discussion ensued that covered Dan's medical condition, his treatment options and their risks and benefits, and his capacity and preferences (he was unresponsive).

When the discussion moved to the next steps, the health care team recommended that the dialysis be discontinued, with efforts shifting to keeping Dan comfortable. The son did not budge from his insistence that his father continue to receive dialysis.

In the days following the ethics consult, the son's minister came to the hospital. He found the patient's son in his father's room, and the two of them began to visit and talk. During their conversation, the son came to the realization that his father was suffering. He asked the nurse to notify the physician that he wanted to talk about his father's care.

When the physician arrived, the son said that he had changed his mind. He could see that his father was suffering. He was ready to request that the dialysis be discontinued. The physician responded empathically to the son, assuring him that Dan would be kept comfortable and that the family could be present. The son got in touch with the rest of the family, asking them to come to the hospital.

With the family present, the health care team disconnected Dan from the dialysis equipment and removed it from the room, which provided more space and also created a more hospitable setting. The patient's son and other members of the family gathered around the patient. Gradually and peacefully, Dan's life came to an end.

The news of the son's decision spread quickly among those involved in Dan's care. They were surprised at this change of mind and were curious about the conversation held by the minister and the son. They were relieved and grateful for Dan: at least his suffering had ended. They were grateful for them-selves and their colleagues. No longer were they required to perform care that only extended suffering.

COMING TO TERMS WITH DEATH: A THRESHOLD FOR HEALERS AND PATIENTS ALIKE

When patients realize that their situation is one of approaching death, they may respond in a variety of ways. There are those patients who do not see death as a failure or as a defeat. Rather, in some instances, there are those patients who view death as a threshold. Death for these patients is no longer a feared enemy, but a welcome relief. They see death as offering peace, rest, and release. It frees the patient from suffering's grip, as can no other means. Additionally, families, given the patient's health circumstances, modify their outlook on death from something to be avoided at all costs to something that can provide peace and release.

Certainly, other patients and their families may sense defeat or manifest fury in the face of death. However, given the meaning structure, spiritual orientation, philosophic outlook, or religious belief of a particular patient and his or her family and the nature and circumstances of the patient's death, death may be viewed as a transition, not a termination. Our culture in the West, and particularly in the United States, avoids dealing with death. This avoidance of facing the inevitability of death is revealed in the attitude that sees death as an option, not a given. Patients and families who view death as an option are more likely to be despondent or furious than those who have come to terms with death as being part of life.

Our present-day funeral observances make efforts to deny the finality of death. Such efforts are seen in the preparation of the body for viewing, the sheets of artificial grass that cover the grave's dirt, the lack of rituals for grieving, and the expectation that people "get over their sorrow" and "get on with their lives." Within health care itself, death may be seen as a failure or as an enemy to be defeated—more than an essential component of life itself. Try as we may to avoid reality, the truth of the matter is that all living things die. Death is not an option.

There are exceptions within subcultures and some religious bodies to this dominant perspective in Western and American culture. Members of these groups have a differing outlook, one where death is viewed as part of life. Within these groups, rituals and practices are in place to support the bereaved as they grieve and honor the death of a loved one. While death certainly causes deep and profound sorrow, some view it as inherent in life, not as an intruder. Death may be seen as coming too soon, or as being a tragedy. Even so, while the timing or the circumstances of a particular death break the family's heart, death in and of itself is acknowledged as one of life's realities.

Unlike our predominant culture, where grief may be viewed as the process for "getting over" the death of a loved one and "moving on" with life, other world cultures cultivate ongoing relationships with deceased loved ones. The dead are honored and revered. They are understood to be present and to have a beneficial influence on their survivors.

For those involved in health care, it is requisite for healers to come to terms with death. Death is a distinct reminder of the finitude of life. Life has a beginning and an end. It is a painful illusion for you to think that death can be beaten or chased away. You will grieve, both as your patient's death approaches and after the actual death itself.

To the extent that you are able to come to terms with the reality of death and appreciate the blessings and benefits it offers for those at the end of life who are suffering intractably, you are likely to find yourself compassionate and peaceful. You will be able to talk with patients and families with a heart sustained by equanimity (balance, harmony). You will be able to comfort their fears and anxieties and listen with sensitivity and empathy to their own views on death and dying. They will sense your openness, kindness, and respect for their feelings, thoughts, observances, and practices.

To whatever degree the patient and family come to terms with death, you will be a comforting and steadying presence. Your healing efforts extend to the surviving loved ones as they begin their journey of grief. Interacting with and relating to you lays the groundwork for a healthy and healing grieving—as much as is possible given the particular dynamics, characteristics, and resources of the individual and his or her family.

The pain in your life is not just a reflection of the pain your patients and their families experience. Your life has its own pain. Part of the human experience is to know joy and sorrow, celebration and dejection. Within the broad spectrum of your pain, the focus of this book is the pain you experience in your role as a healer. What follows is a compelling episode of caring for a clinical colleague and friend. This situation deeply affected multiple healers. What is poignant about this instance is that the care revolved around attending to a friend and colleague who was now a patient—"their" patient.

BECKY'S STORY: SHATTERED DREAMS

Becky had a magnetic personality and a sparkling sense of humor. Her smile was infectious. Her colleagues at the hospital and her friends were drawn to her warmth. It was quite a shock when the news spread that Becky had breast cancer.

Once Becky and her family were through the shock of the diagnosis, she began her treatment. She underwent a mastectomy, chemotherapy, and radiation. During those days, her health care team supported her at home and at work. They took meals to her house and picked up pieces of her job. Becky's supervisor encouraged her to monitor her energy and modify her work schedule accordingly. Through it all, Becky kept her keen wit.

When Becky completed the course of her treatment, no trace of the cancer remained. She had reached the one-mile marker. Her family and her friends at the hospital were ecstatic! Now began the requisite waiting and observations for the next five years.

Finally, she reached the five-year milestone, and her tests continued to show that she was cancer free. Becky could now consider having reconstructive surgery. When she and her family decided that she wanted the surgery, she began to have the necessary workups and examinations. People were encouraging her and happy for her.

During the presurgery preparations, doctors discovered a mass. They ordered more tests, which detected more masses. Her clinical picture now revealed that her cancer had reappeared in an aggressive form. The cancer was so pervasive that there were few, if any, treatment options. Becky's hopes and dreams of undergoing reconstructive surgery were dashed. She now faced a terminal illness and end-of-life care. She and her family were crestfallen—as were her health care team friends and colleagues.

Becky stayed at work as long as her stamina permitted, where she was surrounded by love and compassion. Those on her health care team continued to monitor her condition and did their best to comfort and console her. Her family stood beside her as did her church family.

Becky's multiple healers were so sad. There were no treatment options to pursue. They, too, had shared her initial vision of having the reconstructive surgery, since she had reached and surpassed the five-year anniversary. That goal no longer existed. Becky was now on a different course. The time at hand was for compassion, support, and love.

The reactions among the healers varied. Some hugged her. Some patted her shoulder or back. Some were not able to communicate their affection for her. Others looked into Becky's eyes, saying nothing, while their own eyes watered. Some spoke of their fondness—even love—for her. In their own way, those involved in her care expressed their feelings of love and support. This display of compassion to Becky and her family continued until her death. These expressions were most uplifting to her and her family. They meant more to her than words could say, and they were a great help throughout her decline. Becky died at home, with her family gathered around her.

Much like the healers in this example, you too experience sorrow, irritation, frustration, relief, and happiness as you interact with patients. Quite often, and for a variety of reasons (your training, personality, past observations, and experiences), you may keep your feelings carefully guarded. It is quite likely that you are selective about the people who you open up to. Such individuals are among a trusted few—spouse, partner, valued colleague, medical school professor, residency or fellowship friend. You may think it best to hide your emotions from your patients and your colleagues. It may be your opinion that your sorrow, fear, uncertainty, and anger are to be held in secret as they may be viewed as unprofessional, if not weak.

Certainly, in your interactions with patients, you may think it best to remain professional and somewhat dispassionate for the patients' benefit. Observing professional boundaries is an essential element in providing patient care and in nurturing your self-care.

There is another point of view regarding your emotions, certainly those emotions of compassion, sensitivity, and care. There are those moments when the healing you provide to patients and their families is conveyed through your words, actions, or demeanor. Along those lines, I have witnessed the extraordinary power present when healers show their emotions to patients. I have seen physicians cry with parents whose child died in the emergency room despite every effort to save that child's life. I have seen nurses hug family members who have just heard the physician deliver bad news. I've witnessed caring hands of nurses and physicians placed on the sagging or sobbing shoulders of patients. I have been with respiratory therapists and pharmacists who spoke short sentences of consolation to a patient's family whom they had gotten to know during the course of caring for the patient.

I have been present when chaplains stood in a patient's room with a grieving family, absorbing their sorrow in silence and touching arms or shoulders respectfully and caringly, perhaps with tears in their own eyes. No words—merely a simple touch—a healing touch. After all, what is to be said? Words are often not fitting. More than words, what frequently means the most to patients and families is a caring touch, affectionate facial expressions, or compassionate and loving tears—healing, cleansing tears.

These and other expressions of care, compassion, and empathy heal the hearts of families. Seeing that the physician is not only technically competent and proficient, but also deeply caring about the patient, extends a curative power all its own. When the nurse or the advanced practice clinician values the patient as a person, it often eases the patient's anxiety, lowers the patient's respiration and metabolism rates, slows the patient's heart rate, decreases the patient's blood pressure, and lifts the patient's spirits.

The warmth and kindness of the myriad health care team members who interact with patients and families are all key ingredients in the healing process. Of course it matters that you fulfill your role and responsibilities in a competent manner. At the same time, the soul of everyone involved in patient care—including your soul—transmits and imparts a healing power to the patient.

Actually, while it seems self-evident that emergency situations raise your adrenaline in a physical and figurative manner, it may be less obvious that your soul is touched routinely. You may not be conscious of how often it is moved, as these situations are less dramatic than those in the emergency department.

Nonetheless, there are still powerful and soul-stirring situations that occur through the course of your day. An unexpected spot shows up on a patient's images. A lump is discovered during a patient's routine physical. A sonogram reveals some problems with a fetus. Blood work unexpectedly discloses a major health problem.

How do you as a healer convey such news to a long-time patient or to a patient new to you and your care? How are you emotionally present and caring with a patient and family who are turning over the news in their hearts and minds? What shall be said to the new mother and father concerning what the sonogram reveals about their baby? The healer knows that the patient's anxiety level will elevate when that patient is asked to schedule an office visit to review and discuss the results from diagnostics, such as images, samples, biopsies, or blood work.

These instances are some of the daily heart-touching interactions that wash upon the shore of your soul. Waves of compassion, or suffering with your patients, roll in and roll out. How do you keep going? Where do you find the strength to continue when your body, heart, and mind are pushed to their limits? How you answer this question gets to the source, or wellspring, of your vitality and resiliency.

Sources of Resiliency

Renewing your strength includes two steps: letting go of the burden of the day and renewing your energy for tomorrow. It is important that you have your own ways of putting behind what you experienced today that so profoundly touched you. You may have seen a patient who reminded you of one of your own family members—a grandparent, sibling, or child. You may have seen an improving patient suddenly take a turn for the worse. You may have been in the room with a patient and family who are struggling with the seriousness of the patient's diagnosis. You may have learned of complications being experienced by one of your patients subsequent to the treatment you provided. What are your resources—practices, rituals, and routines—that help you put the past behind you and release you to focus on the present?

Additionally, it is important that you are able to refresh and renew your energy. In the fullest sense, you require rest—of body, mind, and spirit. What are your ways of resting? What rites, rituals, practices, pursuits, and routines bring you distraction, energy, renewal, and freshness? What follows are some suggestions and resources for nurturing and renewing your body, mind, heart, and soul.

PRAYERS, MEDITATIONS, AND REFLECTIONS

On Awakening: No Day Is to Be Taken for Granted, Certainly Not Today

⊟ Ancient Awakener, you who awaken each day with the sun's warmth and light, thanks for my wake-up call this morning. I continue to be amazed that you awaken me. I don't take that lightly. I know that not everybody wakes up from naturally occurring, or medically induced, sleep. My brain must be working because I am praying. My eyes see the clock. My ears hear the coffeemaker brewing. My nose sniffs that coffee's wonderful aroma. This day is brand new. Open my eyes and ears to the marvels and fascinations simply waiting for me to enjoy them. Amen.

For the Gift of the Unexpected: The Disbeliever's Prayer

⊟ I can't believe what happened today. He/she was different! Nice—not nasty. Maybe I changed—maybe I had the wrong picture of that person. It doesn't matter if I changed or if he/she changed; it's still wonderfully unbelievable! Amen.

A Prayer for Healing

⊟ Sacred Soul Searcher, take my pain away. The image of my suffering patient stays with me. There are few, if any, with whom I can discuss my distress. I stood by her bed, knowing full well that I was powerless to stop her decline. Oh, I did things—listened to her respiration and her heart. I felt her pulse and looked at the monitors. I reviewed her chart. Sure, it gave the family and the patient the impression that I was helping. Actually, what I did was for my peace of mind.

Help me see what I did from a different perspective, the view that acknowledges the value of my presence. As I went through those typical and routine gestures, I touched my patient. I spoke to her. I communicated my care for her. While I was in the room, I made it clear that she was important, that her life mattered to me. I spoke with the family. I gave them my attention. I said words of kindness and respect. I offered assurance to the patient and family that I was doing all I could to keep her comfortable and to ensure her dignity.

What I had to offer this patient was me—my heart, my soul, my compassionate presence. Help me always to be amazed and in awe of the healing power of my person and presence. In so doing, may I be blessed with some peace of mind and some healing of my own heart and soul. Amen.

Death: Enemy or Friend?

Source of All Life, you have implanted in us a remarkable will to live. Yet, patients die. Infants, children, adolescents, adults, the elderly—they all succumb to illness or injury. I am the one who is supposed to bar the door and keep away the enemy—death. Sometimes I succeed. Sometimes I cannot stem death's onslaught. Isn't that my job?

Death is not the enemy. Death is part of life. We are born. We die. Death may be sad, even tragic and unfair. Death is not about my discipline or about me as a healer. Everyone dies: the only questions are when and how.

Free me from the illusion, if not egotism, that I can

defeat death. At best, I can postpone it for a later time. On other occasions, I may be able to ease the dying process and death itself. My responsibility is to do what I can within the limits of my discipline, the patient's own state, and the power of the disease or injury. What more can I ask of myself?

Yes, death brings sorrow. That sorrow is deeper and more intense with the young or with an unexpected and tragic onset. In some instances, death marks the graceful end of a life well lived. It is a fitting conclusion. At times, it offers release and relief from an irreversible and inalterable decline and demise. It is a path to peace. Grant me a heart and eye of discernment that I may see the many faces of death. Amen.

Rediscover Your Passion, Purpose, Resiliency

THIS CHAPTER LOOKS closely at the invaluable role passion plays in healing. Passion is presented as the energy that sustains and invigorates health professionals' courage and perseverance, both of which are called upon time and again given the stress they encounter as healers.

Passion is also presented as the driving force that enlivens health care professionals' sense of purpose. Purpose is one of the key elements grounded in the healers' spiritual experience of the Transcendent Source of Life.

Healers know all too well the moments of apprehension and challenge that momentarily dampen and, given the magnitude of the situation, even deplete their passion. Nurture and renewal of passion are vital to health care professionals' resilience. Four sources for that nurture and renewal are: (1) the healers' patients, (2) the healers' particular team, (3) the health care organization in which the health care professionals work, and (4) the self-care healers extend to themselves.

Here I present spiritually based self-care as the most important source of renewal and ongoing nurture for the health care professionals' passion. I will discuss and present specific recommendations for self-care for a healer to consider and implement.

PASSION AS ENERGY

You have a zest for the art and science of healing. Healing ignites a fire in you. A related term for passion is the word *enthusiasm*. In its literal translation, enthusiasm means "in" (en) "God" (theos). Passion entails high spirits and an eagerness and delight in the task at hand.

Health care pulls you to it, drawing you into its gravity field. There is an irresistible attraction for you to be involved in health care. Your passion pulls on you as the moon pulls on the seas.

In health care, you certainly encounter and experience times of discouragement and moments of disillusionment that momentarily flatten and diminish your passion. These moments generally are short-lived. You recover from the setback and find that your passion returns to its typical level. Given the reality that you do experience discouragement, it is essential that you establish patterns and practices for nurturing and cultivating your passion. The processes of nurture and cultivation are known as *self-care*. Such self-care is central to your perseverance in the physically, emotionally, intellectually, and spiritually demanding and draining world of healing. To remain in health care over the long haul, you will be wise to treasure and protect your self-care.

If you neglect your passion, and certainly if a significant event affects your enthusiasm, it is quite possible that you will see a decline in your energy. Such attrition generally occurs over time, a slow but steady decrease in your zeal for healing and for being a healer. You may sense that you are less interested or less satisfied for some reason or another in health care. It may strike you as a malaise that seems to have no specific origin, or you may well be able to isolate an event or series of events as the probable cause.

The continuation of this gradual loss of enthusiasm evolves into *apathy*. Apathy is the absence, or at least an extraordinarily low level of interest (read "passion"), in being a healer. Literally, the word is "a-pathos"—without passion, energy, or drive. When feeling apathetic, you simply begin not to care about contending with all the challenges present day in and day out in health care. You may begin to wonder if you are in the right field. The thrill is gone. You may find that you are dragging yourself to work, that you are giving yourself pep talks for motivation. The days become filled with drudgery. You find yourself wondering quite often, "What am I doing with my life?" With the onset of apathy, this question turns into an existential emptiness, almost an unspoken moan. It becomes a lament, a symptom telling you that you have become disenchanted with health care and your role in it.

Left unaddressed, this state of indifference can worsen, moving to cynicism. With apathy, you are apt to be withdrawn, quiet, and distant from your family, friends, and colleagues—even your patients. Should cynicism set in, you may find yourself angry, bitter, antagonistic, and irritable. Try as you may, the churning of your heart and soul cannot be concealed. Your state of mind, and the condition of your heart, will be revealed in your behavior, interactions, speech, facial expressions, gestures, and the inflection and intensity of your voice. Those around you will be aware of your condition, wondering what is happening to you. They may well speculate if somehow they said or did something displeasing to you.

Your patients will certainly sense your bitterness and irritability. Your speech may be curt. Patients will notice that you are being short, that you brush off their concerns. They will hear the impatience in your voice and your displeasure with them for not getting it or for not satisfactorily cooperating in their care.

Similarly, your colleagues will wonder, "What is wrong with him/her—she/he has become so unpleasant!" Initially, they will be somewhat empathetic, attributing your current state to problems beyond the work place. They grant you the consideration that you are experiencing family or marital problems or that a loved one is in poor health. Eventually it will become clear that something is eating at you, that you are unpleasant to be around, and that you are certainly hard to work with. You will sense their guardedness and distance, which will further exacerbate your pain.

Apathy is not permanent or irreversible. There is hope for you. Apathy and even cynicism are treatable, reversible, and responsive to interventions. Your passion can be renewed. Early detection and self-diagnosis of the initial stages of apathy and cynicism are possible. Listening to loved ones and trusted colleagues who care enough about you to ask, "What is going on with you?" can be an encouragement to you to address your current state. When those you trust say, "You do not seem happy," they do so on the basis of your best interest. Brushing off such demonstrations of care for you with comments like "nothing" or "I am fine" will only make your apathy worse. If you are able to absorb the expressions of care for you, then you will be able to address your loss of zeal early in its appearance. As you well know, early intervention is far and above preferable and more effective than that of playing catch up when apathy and cynicism are full blown.

Some health care professionals do discover that health care is not for them. It neither offers the rewards nor the satisfaction they envisioned. Such a realization and recognition may well serve you. After all, you have many gifts. There are other careers you may pursue. There are other outlets for your creativity, your ability to learn, and your desire to make a difference.

Be kind to yourself. You are not under a mandate to be a healer—no "shoulds" or "oughts" obligate you to pursue and persist in a health care career. What does matter is that you invest your life in what you want to do, what makes you happy, what puts a smile on your face, and what warms your heart. Restated, within you resides the cure for what ails you. Within you are the resources for restoring yourself to a state of well-being—a harmony of body, mind, and spirit in which you experience an elevation and renewal of your passion for life—*your* life.

What follows is an amazing story of a person who fled to the United States to save his life and that of his children. His wife had been killed in his nation's upheaval. If anyone had occasion to have lost their passion, this man fit the criteria.

Randy's Story:
Keep Your Eyes on the Prize

Randy's nation was in the grips of armed conflict, conflict that had claimed the life of his wife and the lives of many of his friends. Randy knew that he and his children were in danger so he sought the safety of the United States. With the help of sponsors, he and his two sons immigrated to the United States where he could begin a new life.

He arrived with little more than the clothes on his back and what could be carried in a suitcase. He had lost his native land, his wife, and his culture. He had not lost his zeal.

Randy's English was elementary at best, which limited his employment options. He finally landed a job as a nurse's aide in a local hospital. Now he had a steady income and health insurance. He and his children were able to get their own apartment. He enrolled his children in school. Things were looking up.

At work, Randy had the opportunity to work on his English. He took advantage of English as a second language classes offered by the hospital. His workmates and colleagues in the hospital also coached and encouraged him.

Randy worked closely with the nurses and saw the importance of their role. He saw them interact with patients and their families. He admired their professional knowledge and skills. It dawned on Randy that he wanted to be a nurse! He wondered how he could possibly accomplish that goal. He was a single parent. He was making minimum wage. His English was limited.

One day, Randy voiced his dream to one of his nurse friends. Much to Randy's amazement, the nurse encouraged him. The nurse told him that the hospital had a program to help people attend nursing school. The nurse assured Randy that he could work and attend classes. It would take time and effort, but Randy could do it.

Inspired by his dream, and equipped with the knowledge his nurse friend provided, Randy enrolled in nursing school. Today, Randy is a nurse, working at a hospital. His passion for health care gave a him a new world and a new life.

You have your own story of how you became passionate about health care. Over the years, that initial spark may have increased as you found yourself more and more excited by what you were doing as a healer. When you find yourself sagging, your spirits low, call to mind that early spark. It may yet have the power to reignite your passion's fire.

Self-Care

Healers have an ethical obligation to exercise self-care. This ethic may strike you as being antithetical to the ethic of caring for others. However, these two obligations are actually complimentary. The dictum "do no harm" clearly applies to patients for whom you care about. It also applies to you! To put the above instruction into a positive statement, the phrase "seek well-being" applies to your patient care and to your self-care.

The ratio of risk and benefit also points to the importance of your self-care. There is a culture of being a hero, of showing super-human stamina, commitment, and devotion to patients. There is certainly applause for those healers who put patients first to the extent that they sacrifice their rest and their time with family and friends. This applause can drown out words of caution regarding this pace.

Healing itself recognizes the risk of not allowing time for rest and rejuvenation. Working long and hard hours takes its toll. That toll may include harm to intimate relationships at home with your partner and children. The toll may be the harm to friendships. Not allowing or requiring yourself to rest poses risks to your patients. Tired, if not fatigued, healers must make decisions and perform interventions when their mind is not as sharp and their hand not as steady. Healers, their patients, their colleagues, and their loved ones all benefit when the healer observes self-care.

Self-care may sound like something else you have to do. Actually, self-care is not something else. Self-care is woven into the rhythm of your life. When you are not scheduled to work, turn off your pager. Do not check your messages—text messages, e-mails, voice messages. When you are off duty, you are off! Your trusted and competent colleagues are seeing to patient care.

When you are at work, self-care may be as simple as stepping into the break room. You often walk down a hall with windows. Look outside. Take in the light, the sky, the horizon. You may cross paths with a friend. Say hello. You may even have a few moments to ask about his or her weekend. These examples are but a few of the ways where you can find a way to tend to your spirit. Lift your nose up from the grindstone, and you will be surprised and delighted at the opportunities to get a breath of fresh air over the course of a day.

Self-care can be as simple as companionship. What follows is the story of two nurses on a pediatric floor who responded to an unexpected death.

Wanda's Story: The Power of Being a Companion

One night, there was an unexpected death on the pediatrics floor. The child, a preschooler named Roy, had been a patient in the pediatric intensive care unit and had improved sufficiently to be moved to the general pediatrics floor. His parents felt confident enough with their son's improved condition to go home for the night. A night of rest was long overdue as they had been spending extended hours at the hospital.

Wanda was a new graduate from nursing school and excited to have her first job, particularly in pediatrics. She was working the night shift and was glad to have Paula with her on the floor as Paula was an experienced nurse.

The patients were asleep. All seemed well. Wanda made

her scheduled rounds, stepping into each room to check on her patients. Entering Roy's room, she approached his bed. Wanda noticed how still Roy was. She looked more closely. He was not breathing. She quickly took his pulse. There was no pulse, and his skin was cool to her touch.

Wanda immediately pushed the code blue alarm and called for Paula. They began CPR on Roy, stepping back with the arrival of the code blue team. The health care team placed a phone call to the parents, requesting them to come to the hospital as quickly as possible. The code blue team members worked on Roy but were unable to revive him. When they called the code and the CPR activities ended, everyone left the room sad.

Roy's parents lived some distance from the hospital and had not arrived yet at the hospital. Wanda needed to prepare Roy's body and room for his parents' visit. Paula knew that Roy's death was the first patient death for Wanda. Paula could see the sorrow and strain on Wanda's face as Wanda prepared Roy's body and arranged his bed. Paula said, "Want me to help?" Wanda nodded, "Yes."

While Roy's parents arrived and spent time with their son, Wanda and Paula sat at the nurses' station. They were both quiet. After a bit, Wanda looked at Paula and said, "Thanks."

Every healer has his or her first patient death. That death is a mile marker in a healer's career. Paula realized the impact of this death, empathized with Wanda, and gently offered support—the support of being present. Wanda did not attempt to display bravado or assume an "I can take it" posture. She accepted Paula's offer and, in doing so, exercised self-care. Wanda's self-care was not an add on. Rather, in the midst of accomplishing what had to be done in preparation for the arrival of Roy's parents, she cared for herself by having Paula present.

You, too, are able to care for yourself at the same time you are fulfilling your patient care duties. Self-care is as simple as having the presence of someone who understands.

PATIENTS AS RECHARGERS

Among the multiple ways you are able to boost your passion, patients are second only to your intimate relationships—family, friends, trusted others—as a powerful well from which you may draw waters of rejuvenation. It is easy to conceive of the healer-patient relationship as one-sided: the healer is the provider of health care, and the patient is the recipient.

You know from your own experience that your interaction with patients is actually a two-way process. Both you and your patients give and receive. In fact, patients are perhaps one of the most powerful replenishers of your passion! They give you a charge and, not infrequently, recharge your ebbing energy.

How do patients lift your spirits and renew your passion? They do so in simple and everyday ways. They smile at you. They express how much they appreciate you. They convey their gratitude for what you are doing and have done for them. They shake your hand and may even give you a hug!

Such patients are gifts. In contrast, there are numerous patients who are energy drains. They are full of complaints. They are unhappy with you and with their care in general. They appreciate very little that you do or recommend, and your efforts are rarely well received. You know them well. Interacting with them requires a great deal of emotional energy as you work to remain respectful, calm, courteous, and attentive to their complaints—if not outright attacks on you and your competency! You may pause to take a breath and collect yourself before you step into the exam room where such patients await you.

The drain on your energy by these patients can outweigh the encouragement you receive from appreciative and kind patients, which is all the more reason to recognize and absorb what your energizing patients offer. It is a mystery how negative comments and criticism appear to hold more power than compliments and words of gratitude. See what you can do to reverse that order. It does not have to be that way.

Hold the grateful and appreciative patients in your heart and memory. You can recall such patients to act as an antibiotic and antidote to the deflation inflicted by the power-draining patients. Practice calling them to mind over the course of the day, especially when you find the voice of the complaining patient sounding in your head. Let your grateful patients show this complainer the door! Your appreciative patients far outnumber your complaining patients. Let their collective voice drown out the complaints of your unappreciative patients.

A Grandmother's Story: Adding to the Family

The health care team paged the chaplain on call to visit a patient who had requested one. When the chaplain arrived, he found an elderly Navajo patient. Her adult granddaughter sat by her bed. The chaplain introduced himself to the patient and to the granddaughter, saying that he understood that they wanted to see a chaplain. The granddaughter spoke, explaining that her grandmother did not speak English. She said that her grandmother wanted a Bible. The chaplain replied that he would be glad to get a Bible and excused himself from the room.

Returning with the Bible, he smiled at the patient and at her granddaughter. He gave the Bible to the granddaughter, who then handed it to her grandmother. They visited a bit, with the granddaughter helping the chaplain talk to her grandmother by interpreting for the two of them—from English to Navajo and from Navajo to English. After a while, the chaplain said good-bye and left the room.

Later in the day, the chaplain received a page back to the same room. When he arrived, he learned the patient's medicine man was present, and the patient wanted the chaplain to join them in her room. The granddaughter explained to the chaplain that her grandmother was adopting him as one of her "sons." The chaplain was speechless. The patient was smiling at him. He asked the granddaughter to tell her grandmother how deeply touched and honored he was. The granddaughter interpreted his comments. The patient extended her hand to the chaplain, who took her hand in his. As they held one another's hands, she spoke to her granddaughter. When the granddaughter interpreted, she said that her grandmother wanted him to add his prayers to those of the medicine man. The chaplain was speechless. What a heartwarming moment.

Every healer has his or her own similar story, a story of a patient, or a patient's family, who made a lasting impression. These moments are gifts. These patients stay with you, living in your memory and visiting you on occasion to remind you of the difference you make, which is often unknown to you and in the midst of doing what you ordinarily do. Except, for this patient, your "ordinary" action was a course-changer in his or her hospital stay.

Patients also lift your spirits as you see your intervention and care bring them benefit. More often than not, what you do brings relief and healing to your patients. Your sense of accomplishment and rightful pride in your healing competencies and successes both give you a boost. Not only do you see the good you have provided for your patients, you experience professional and personal satisfaction in your ability to help others. Self-affirmation is important. You know that you are good at what you do. In your health care career, you will have the gift and blessing of seeing growth and improvement in your practice of healing. You will see that you are becoming better—how satisfying!

Sometimes your efforts afford little or no help to patients or do not reach the level of outcome that you expected and hoped would be attained. When that happens, you attempt a new track. When you conclude that the level of improvement that can be achieved has been reached, then you accept that fact. You can take some degree of professional pride in that you did help the patient achieve what was possible under the circumstances.

Beyond the gift of recharging your passion that your patients grant, there are other ways for you to replenish it. Call to mind what restores and sustains your passion for your career. What part does the appreciation of your colleagues and coworkers play in keeping your passion alive? What energy do you draw from attending professional development functions, reading, pursuing hobbies, exercising, resting, and nurturing your soul with prayer, meditation, reflection, solitude, and silence?

Are you paying attention to your family? Do you appreciate

how your partner, spouse, children, and relatives value your passion? A few pages ago, I said that patients were the secondary source of rejuvenation for your spirits, with your intimate relationships being primary and of utmost importance. It is tempting to see how much your patients need you. But your family needs you more than your patients! You need your family and their encouragement and understanding more than you need the satisfaction found in patient care. Watch out for saying that you spend quality time with your family while diminishing quantity time. Quality and quantity are inseparable. The depth of relationships also includes duration. Quality is the blossom of a relationship built over time. Taking the time for your family—attending your children's school and extracurricular activities, watching them at recitals and sports events, being present for their birthday parties, planning family outings—is important for the health of those relationships and for the mutual well-being of you and your family.

Taking the time—being at home and being present when you are home—for your spouse or significant other matters. Being present means no phone calls, no texts, no e-mail—all of which take your attention and presence away from your loved ones. Doing simple things with your loved ones, such as going for walks, watching movies at home, planning a night out, supporting their interests and pursuits, or listening as they talk to you about what is going on with their lives, are all mutually enriching. These and other expressions demonstrate and communicate your affection for those who love and esteem you.

The love of your family and spouse or significant other is your breath, your heartbeat, and your balance and harmony. Treasure and nurture these relationships. Nothing else matters as much nor is of greater value.

Your Team: Energizing or Exhausting?

Passion also involves your broader work setting and culture. The health care organization in which you serve as a healer can be a passion extinguisher or a passion igniter. Your team—section, practice, unit, floor—can be a toxin or a tonic.

Passion feeds and builds on passion. Call it team spirit. Call it team pride. The positive spirit of a team is conducted and transmitted among and within the team, energizing the team members—including you. In like fashion, the reverse is true in a setting rife with animosity, friction, and "me first" thinking. You are not immune to the ill health of your team and organization.

Be kind to yourself. Value yourself. Some soil simply will not support plant life. It is too depleted. Find a team and a culture that make you excited about what they are doing for their patients.

It may take a while to get a read on the pulse of your team. You may be excited and pleased to see the commitment and competence of your colleagues. Or, you may be disappointed—if not dismayed—to learn of the low spirits and inferior quality of patient care.

When you do make this discovery, be honest with yourself. A healthy team will stay that way only as long as the team members commit themselves to working at keeping their interactions supportive and encouraging. Sharing common goals, communicating clearly and in a timely fashion, clarifying misunderstandings, resolving differences, and being forgiving and tolerant are the features that nourish and sustain a healthy team spirit.

A vital team establishes an environment where recognition is granted and received. The atmosphere is one of excitement. Creativity and innovation are present, encouraged, and invited. Each team member senses that he or she is contributing to the mission of the team in a way that is personally fulfilling. Team members are valued for their individual gifts and for how they contribute in a synergistic way to the accomplishments of the team as it does its part in providing patient care.

Patients sense your passion as well as that of the broader health care team. Passion transmits a healing energy to patients. They can remind you that you like what you do, that you are excited to be a healer, and that you feel your role allows you to make a difference in the lives of those for whom you care.

At the same time, patients pick up on diminished passion. They see it in your face. They hear it in your voice. They feel it in your touch. You are not happy. Something is on your mind. Your attention is elsewhere, which detracts from your being present and being compassionate with this particular patient.

Humor is one way a team keeps up its energy level. A humorless team is likely to be a low-energy team. One nurses' team knew how to laugh with each other. Here is a story about how the power of humor kept up a team's energy.

AMY'S STORY: *Saturday Night Live*

During a recent presidential campaign, *Saturday Night Live* was doing its usual parody and impersonation of various candidates. One of the unit charge nurses had an amazing ability to mimic those routines, much to the amusement of the varied health care professionals who happened by her.

This nurse's uncanny comic ability was admired, and people would egg her on to do an impersonation. The smiles and energy she evoked were contagious. Given the patient acuity on that floor and the heaviness that frequently was present, her humor was a welcome relief and a much-needed source of energy.

The cohesion of this team and their job satisfaction was evident. The team members were cooperative and considerate of one another. Patients and families sensed that their nurses were glad to be there. Others in the hospital who had reason to come to the unit could feel the energy in the air. Who are those people on your team who pick up your spirits? They are there.

The Organization as Biosphere

Your team exists within a larger system, which is the health care organization itself. The organization, composed of multiple systems and subsystems, is the biosphere for your team and the organization's other teams and components. What you and your team require is that your organization's biosphere be invigorating, literally and figuratively. Passion thrives in those organizations that have a clear vision, a stirring mission, sound values, and dedication to providing excellent patient care. You and your team look for support and appreciation from the organization for your contributions to patient care.

Here is an instance when the sensitive action by leadership was both comforting and encouraging.

Claudia's Story: Bearing One Another's Sorrow

Claudia said good-bye to her family and got into her car to travel to the retreat center for the organization's system-wide meeting. While at the meeting, she received a message to call her husband at home. What she heard was a lightning bolt from the blue. He was calling to tell her the devastating news of their son's tragic death. He was involved in a one-car accident and died at the scene.

Somehow, Claudia found her way back to the meeting room. She went to her supervisor and asked him to step into the hall. He knew from the look on Claudia's face that something awful had happened. In the hall, she told him of her son's death and her need to go home. The supervisor went into high gear. He rounded up other members of the team. The team made plans for two people to drive Claudia home so that she was safe and supported.

Next, the supervisor approached the senior leadership team members to alert them to this crisis. The senior leadership team was shocked and saddened as they listened to the supervisor relate the tragedy that had befallen Claudia and her family. They expressed their sympathies and requested that the supervisor tell Claudia they would support her and her family through this sorrow.

The senior leadership team realized that this tragedy would affect the facility where this team worked. It was a small facility in a small town. The staff at that facility were close knit; they were friends and neighbors as well as colleagues. The senior leadership team arranged for the organization's critical incident stress management team to go that facility to provide support.

During a break in the retreat's agenda, the CEO spoke to the gathered leaders and team members. He told them of the tragedy that had struck Claudia and her family, asking the audience to keep Claudia and her family in their hearts and prayers.

He outlined the steps he and the senior leadership team had taken to comfort and support Claudia. He acknowledged the impact that this sorrow would have on the facility and said that he had requested the crisis intervention team to travel to that community and facility. He ended his remarks by saying that he would update the attendees as he had further word.

Everyone was shocked and saddened. In the midst of that disbelief and sorrow was deep appreciation for the way that the organization had promptly and compassionately responded. The team was grateful for the support extended to Claudia, her family, and her workmates. It made them proud to be part of such a caring organization.

By these acts of kindness, the organization put a human face on the senior leadership team—certainly the CEO. These and similar expressions of human warmth are of incalculable worth across the organization. Working in health care is stressful and demanding. When members of that organization sense that they are valued and respected as individuals, and not simply as "workers," they manage the stress and demands far better.

A supportive and encouraging upper-level leadership puts the entire organization at ease and creates a sense of common goals being sought through combined and coordinated efforts. When you observe unclear and intermittent communications, experience abrupt changes, or begin to sense that you and your colleagues are not valued, it becomes difficult to be upbeat and energized.

Particularly in these days of seismic, sweeping changes in how health care is provided and funded, uncertainty is a stark reality for any health care organization, as well as its staff and employees.

You and your team are affected by this uncertainty. While the organization makes its own efforts to contend with political and economic powers largely beyond its influence, you need your own resources for living with this uncertainty on a daily basis. Fear and anxiety are close by, watching for an opening to take up occupancy in your thinking and feelings.

Hope, courage, and the "one day at a time" mindset will serve you well. Your passion for what you do and your deeply imbedded awareness that you are making a difference in the lives of those patients you are privileged to serve are essential in the face of this constant stress. Do your best to stay in the moment, and focus on the tasks at hand. Wishing things were otherwise within your specific team or organization will not help.

Thankfully, there are healthy teams that manage, navigate, and survive the inevitable rough spots. They are committed to one another, to the quality of their service, and to their patients. Hopefully, your team possesses these qualities. Above all, remember—you have options. Grant yourself the freedom to evaluate the health of your team and organization. If your team is relatively healthy, you are blessed. If you team is tension filled and with low morale, you may want to find a setting where you are happier and more fulfilled. Be careful in this quest. The grass is not always greener on the other side of the fence. The stresses, strains, and uncertainty within health care are pervasive. At the same time, life is too short for you to be constantly dissatisfied, with no improvement on the horizon. Be good to yourself.

Fear and Anxiety

Healers often stand eye to eye with fear and anxiety. Earlier, our conversation touched on the fear and anxiety generated by the far-reaching changes underway in our nation regarding the availability, provision, and funding of health care. The marketplace, the ballot box, regulatory bodies, and the executive, legislative and judicial branches of government are formidable sources of uncertainty and apprehension in the world of health care.

There is much in healing that merits fear apart from politics and economics. Health care itself is fraught with danger, threat, and peril. Some of the danger is to you as a healer—needle sticks, exposure to infection prior to it being identified, and other forms of contamination. Beyond sticks, spills, and infection, the danger may be your personal safety. Patients or family members are known to lash out at you verbally and, at times, physically. Violence in the workplace is not limited to just patients and families, as individuals with a grudge, or who are unhappy or jealous, are also real and potential sources of violence.

You have enough experience and awareness to expect the unexpected. Patients can faint, fall, go into shock, have an anaphylactic reaction, begin to bleed, develop an irregular heartbeat, stop breathing, or have a sudden heart arrest. You are mindful that successful health care, and a satisfactory conclusion to providing health care, is never to be taken for granted. You know that a little caution goes a long way in the world of health care.

Another ever-present peril and apprehension is the threat of litigation. You as a healer have a lot on the line when it comes to lawsuits: your income, license, certification, and privileges are jeopardized. Suits against healers, and against their employers (organizations have the deep pockets, not you), are commonplace. We've all seen commercials by lawyers and law firms seeking plaintiffs, those persons wishing to bring a personal injury lawsuit against a healer. You live with the realization that you can be sued, a time-consuming and energy-depleting process.

Risk is always present in providing health care. There is no treatment or procedure that is ever "routine." You may refer to an intervention or procedure as routine, meaning that you have experience with it and have performed it countless times. You may employ the term as your way of putting the patient at ease. You are communicating that the patient's situation is not that unusual and that relief and recovery are within reach.

Simultaneously, you know that most patient care, including medications, procedures, or even being in the hospital itself where opportunistic infections stalk the halls in search of a new host, has a greater or lesser degree of risk. An unremarkable procedure is always a cause for gratitude for patient and healer alike.

WALLY'S STORY: HOW DID THAT HAPPEN?

Wally's patient was brought up from the recovery room. Her surgery had gone well. Wally helped get the patient settled in her room and then left for a moment to get her medications. Wally read the orders, got the prescribed medication from the secure medication cart, and filled a syringe with the ordered dosage.

He went back to the patient and administered the medication. He waited a few moments, checked the IVs, and left to do his charting. The patient's husband was in the room, watching his wife sleep. Shorty he noticed that she was not breathing. He got up and gently shook her shoulder—no response. He went to the doorway and shouted, "Nurse!"

Wally and other nurses were there in an instant. They immediately called the code blue team, which was there in a flash. As the husband stood in the corner of the room, the team worked to resuscitate his wife. Wally went to the husband and escorted him to the patient conference room. The health care team paged the chaplain and, on arriving, guided the chaplain to the patient's husband. They sat silently, waiting to hear some news.

When the physician knocked and entered the room, the patient's husband looked at him hopefully. The physician sat down and said that they had not been able to resuscitate his wife. He asked if the husband had any questions. "What happened?" he replied. The physician said that they were not certain at this time but were looking into what happened. He assured the husband that as information became available, they would pass that on to him. Offering his condolences, the physician left the room.

In the nurses' break room, Wally and others involved in caring for this patient were in shock. As their minds wondered, "How could this be?" they were certain that this event would be treated as a sentinel event. A review would be conducted, encompassing every step in the care of this patient and everyone who had a hand in her care.

This "routine" surgery became a tragic sorrow. A husband lost his wife. The staff grieved for him and was in disbelief. They knew that each step would be reviewed: from the operating room to recovery, from the pharmacy to the medication cart, from the physician's order to the nurse's syringe.

A good many of you have an appreciation for this situation, one you have experienced personally or one that has affected a colleague. These moments require you to have in place those people to whom you can turn: people who will honor your confidentiality and who will share their wisdom. These trusted others respect the apprehension, if not fear, that you may be experiencing in the wake of an event like this.

From the patient's perspective, no treatment is routine. Typically, patients are unaccustomed to having a health problem. Good health is routine for them, not illness or injury—apart from the chronically ill who have faced health challenges for a good part of their lives. Going about their lives is routine—not being in your office or the clinic. The treatment scheduled for them is foreign, probably the first time they have been on this medication or required that intervention. Even though what you are recommending or providing to the patient holds the promise of a return to their daily activities, the patient experiences some degree of apprehension.

Patient education is invaluable and answers a good many of your patients' questions. Being open to the patients' questions and concerns will help ease their minds. I suggest that you acknowledge and affirm their anxieties. It may seem counterintuitive, if not ill advised, to ask your patients about what worries or concerns them or the family. Providing a setting where your patients sense your concern and understanding of their unique apprehensions actually strengthens their confidence and trust in you. You can assure the patient that what is on his or her mind is fairly typical and common to other patients and that you respect those fears and feelings. With their concerns out on the table, you have an opportunity to provide information, education, encouragement, and assurance. Ask your patients if you are answering all their questions. They will be grateful and certainly more at ease.

COURAGE: A KEY TO RESILIENCY

To be a healer requires a certain temperament. One aspect of this temperament is the courage to contend with fear and anxiety. You may not see yourself as particularly courageous. Yet, you are a courageous person! Courage is one of your many gifts. Yes, you have the gifts of intellect, aptitude, and compassion, all of which are prerequisites to becoming a healer. Courage is also a prerequisite.

You know full well the dangers and threats inherent in health care. You bring your own fears and anxieties with you. Think for a moment of the everyday instances that require courage of you. It requires courage to see a patient waiting to learn his or her diagnosis, prognosis, and treatment options. It takes courage for you to sit with a patient and discuss a life-threatening, if not life-shortening, illness or injury. It takes courage to enter a patient's room when that patient is anguished, frightened, or coming to terms with the consequences of his or her illness or injury. Courage is demonstrated every time you enter a room where infection control protocols are in place.

Courage is evidenced by your integrity. Whatever your role or discipline, you are guided by your ethics. At the base of your ethics is your particular religious, spiritual, or philosophical understanding of what is good, evil, true, false, constructive, or destructive. You have a frame of reference for what is meaningful and purposeful. To the profound questions about creation itself, the origin of life, the why of death, the wonder of love, the bonds of community, the power of hope, and the horror of chaos, you have understandings and perspectives that steer your daily conduct and interactions.

In addition to your personal ethics, you are guided by the values of the organization itself. These organizational values encompass everyone affiliated with the organization, including governance, senior leadership, administration, volunteers, clinicians, employees, vendors, and contractors. These values define a code of conduct that everyone is expected to honor and follow.

Your ethics likewise are grounded in your particular discipline's professional ethics or code of conduct. It may be that at the completion of your education and training, you were charged to adhere to certain standards. You may have made a promise or taken a vow that you would henceforth fashion your professional life in accordance with certain ethics.

Given your ethics-rich situation, there are many occasions where your courage will prompt you to speak against or speak for a topic under consideration. For instance, at the governance and leadership levels, where there is a mix of administrators, volunteer community members, and clinicians, your ethics may prompt you to support or oppose a particular proposal or action. It takes courage to do so, particularly if you are the sole voice or among the voices of the minority.

With regard to patient care, your ethics may prompt you to advocate for a patient. You may champion for a particular treatment, medicine, or intervention that holds promise and benefits for your patient. Such advocacy may put you at odds with the patient's health plan or with your colleagues who do not agree with you. There are situations where you have to say something about an aspect of patient care (a policy, a process, a practice) that simply strikes you as unethical. You take your concerns and objections to your colleagues and to decision-makers, seeking a review and revision of what has been initiated. Such advocacy is an act of courage. Every time you speak up and out for the patient on the basis of your ethics, you demonstrate courage.

What follows is a story about one physician's courage in following the requests of the patient's health care decision-maker.

SIMON'S STORY: COURAGE UNDER PRESSURE

Simon was born with developmental disabilities and had been medically fragile all his life. Now as a middle-aged adult, his health care decision-maker was Luke. Given Simon's medical conditions, aspiration was a constant threat. Due to his recurring aspiration, Simon had been admitted repeatedly to the hospital. Luke was always present, attending to Simon's care and working with the health care team to ensure Simon received the best possible care.

After one such hospital admission, it was clear that Simon's body was running out of the reserves required to meet the challenge of repeated aspirations. When Simon was ready for discharge from the hospital and was being prepared for transportation to a short-term care facility, Luke learned from the health care team precisely how frail and fragile Simon was. Luke could see it. He knew Simon well. What the healers were describing only confirmed what he sensed.

At the short-term care facility, Simon continued to decline. Since he was an aspiration risk, the staff took great caution in feeding him by mouth. What he could take in orally was inadequate nutrition to fuel his healing and sustain his life. Luke saw the dilemma: risk feeding Simon by mouth and risk death by aspiration, or reduce his oral feeding to such a low level that Simon's body would not have the nutrients required to sustain life.

Luke requested a conference with the physician about what options were available to Simon. The physician reviewed Simon's situation and said that Simon's only option was a feeding tube. The physician described the insertion of the tube, pointing out that while the feeding tube would provide nutrition, it did nothing to reduce Simon's aspiration risk. Luke questioned the physician, making certain that he fully comprehended Simon's situation. He went home, pondering what to do.

The next day, he found the physician and asked if they could talk. Luke said that he had come to a decision. He did not want a feeding tube for Simon. He wanted Simon to be comfortable.

When community advocates learned of Simon's situation and of Luke's decision, they launched a public protest. Luke was accused of failing to protect Simon, and the physician was assailed as not doing enough. The protesters threatened legal action. Luke assured the physician that he was firm in his decision. The physician honored Luke's decision and did not insert a feeding tube. Doing so subjected him and Luke to public pressure and accusation. The physician demonstrated compassion and courage by his commitment to Luke and care for Simon.

It may not occur to you that you are a person of courage. You may see yourself as simply "doing your job." Extend some recognition to yourself: in addition to your training and experience, you possess courage. Because you are courageous, you are able to utilize your skills and compassion to the greater benefit of your patients.

PERSEVERANCE: RESILIENCE GETS YOU UP WHEN LIFE KNOCKS YOU DOWN

Perseverance is one of your strengths. Health care can deliver hard knocks and blows to your body, mind, and spirit. You are not taking a walk in the park as a healer. Beyond the bumps experienced dealing with difficult colleagues, the expectations of your supervisor, or the requirements of the organization, you occasionally experience a clinical situation that deals you a staggering blow. You will have your passion knocked out of you. Most healers get knocked down over the course of their career. Don't feel alone when it happens to you. What follows is an example of a healer being knocked down.

KEN'S STORY: A "HOT" APPENDIX

A teenage male had been in and out of the emergency department over a period of several days, complaining of a stomachache and having difficulty keeping his food down. Several clinicians saw Ken, and he had multiple diagnostic workups. Nothing showed up. The health care team gave him something for his stomach and sent him home.

Within days, Ken was rushed to the hospital by ambulance, not breathing on his own and without a heartbeat. Efforts to resuscitate the teenager were unsuccessful. The cause of death was determined to be a "hot" appendix that had gone undetected. It ruptured, causing systemic sepsis and, subsequently, the teenager's death. Those clinicians who had seen the patient earlier were shaken at the news of Ken's death.

Healers experience these instances and others like it. When these situations occur, you may doubt your skills. Your self-confidence may be eroded. You play the event over and over in your mind, wondering how "that" happened and how you "missed" something that you always catch. Given the magnitude of the event, the thought may cross your mind that health care is not the place for you. In the above case, professionals experienced deep and persistent doubts about their competence. Their self-confidence was tremendously shaken. They felt responsible, concluding that they had let down this patient.

These and other thoughts and feelings are typical among healers. When events knock you down, be kind to yourself. You are human. Things do not always go according to plan. In spite of all the protocols being followed, all the standards of care being observed, and all the diagnostics, a patient's underlying problem is capable of defying detection. It happens. Sometimes all the proverbial holes in the Swiss cheese line up, and you are the one in the wrong place at the right time.

In the aftermath of such experiences, your spirits may be down for a considerable period of time. Respect the magnitude of such events and their impact on your body, mind, and spirit. It may prove beneficial for you to take some time to recover from the blow you took. Many organizations have wellness or occupational health programs and services where you can seek professional and confidential help. Your community may have trusted and competent behavioral health professionals with whom you can work through such crises. If you become aware of your efforts to self-medicate (alcohol, drugs) or if you notice that your behavior is affected (irritable, forlorn, various forms of acting out), seek professional help promptly.

More often than not—and you may well have had this experience already—you will get back on your feet on your own. You will pick yourself up. Your friends and colleagues will reach out to you and give you a shoulder to lean on as they help lift and steady you. It takes strength to get up. It takes resilience to dust yourself off and step back into patient care. These and other acts of determination are exactly what you do! You resume your role. In doing so, you show your tenacity. Health care is not for the faint of heart. You know that. So give yourself some credit and appreciation for being not only a competent and compassionate healer, but a strong one as well!

PURPOSE: STAYING THE COURSE

It is purpose that fuels your perseverance, courage, and resiliency. Being a healer is your life's purpose—one woven into the very fabric of your being. Cross winds and rough seas will bring stress with their storms, putting your purpose to the test. "Do I really want to do this?" is a question that will pay a visit every so often.

You may tell yourself that you don't make enough money for all the pressure put on you or that the finesse and expertise required to provide excellent health care goes underappreciated by your team or by the organization. You may think it attractive to make less money doing something else that involves less stress and time, thereby allowing you the latitude for personal pursuits and family time.

So, what exactly, does keep you in health care? The answer

to this question resides deep within you. It is in your bones. It courses through your arteries. It is the fire in your belly and the beat in your heart. You worked hard to be where you are, and you will not easily be chased off or pushed away. Health care is more than what you do: it is who you are. You are healer. You may need to find another organization, another practice, another setting in which to pursue your passion. The "where" of your calling is less important than the "what" of your purpose.

Your purpose helps you have a clear focus and a definite direction in your life. Nothing else at the moment can match the fulfillment and satisfaction of what you do and who you are. Your eyes are not drawn to other horizons. You know that other options are out there, vying for your attention. As is sometimes said, it never hurts your diet to look at the desserts on the menu.

You are quite attuned to the shortcomings of your current setting. You know the peculiarities of your colleagues. You know the unpleasant features of your work culture. None of these has the power to dilute your focus or alter the direction of your life. You navigate your life by health care's north star. You may have to trim your sails given the way the wind is blowing, but to do so only serves to keep you on the course you have plotted for your life.

Vincent's Story: There Are Many Roads to Rome

Vincent was an outstanding student in medical school and continued to be a high performer in his residency. Upon completing his residency in internal medicine, he began his career. Given his accomplishments, he came to the attention of a major hospital and was offered an administrative position. He would be leading a team of physicians as they pioneered new models of patient care.

For Vincent, this position was a dream come true. It would give him the opportunity to use his intellect, his leadership, and organizational skills; work with colleagues; and have his hand in patient care. He began his new job with enthusiasm.

The first year or so went fairly well. Vincent felt supported by his supervisors, and his team was doing well with their roles and responsibilities. Gradually, his supervisor became less supportive and enthusiastic about Vincent's initiatives. Vincent found the hesitation and reluctance surprising and did his best to meet that challenge. It became increasingly difficult for Vincent to meet the objections of his supervisor.

What started out as a dream job had now become an ordeal. Vincent was not sleeping well. His days were filled with frustration. His team was losing their enthusiasm as well. The vision held out to them was changing, and in ways that they found unwelcome. Vincent's usual chipper and cheerful demeanor was giving way to disillusionment. Vincent began to question his judgment, his present position, and even his career as a physician.

Vincent realized that there was life beyond his current position, and began to consider other options. What he found was a position with an internal medicine practice group. The position offered him less pressure, a positive group of peers, and more patient contact. He and his wife weighed his options, and agreed that reentering private practice was a good move for him and for the family.

He accepted the job and threw himself into seeing patients. He discovered a renewal of his energy and a growing professional satisfaction as he cared for his patients. A smile returned to his face.

PRAYERS, MEDITATIONS, AND REFLECTIONS

When the Flame Flickers

⌐ Fire Starter, you who ignited the stars and our sun, my fire needs stoking, if not relighting. I look at the stars and envy their fire. I look at creative and enthusiastic people and mourn the ashes lodged in my heart. You are the one who first sparked my passion to be a healer. Be merciful and compassionate as my coals burn low. Restore my faltering passion. Fill me with zeal and zest. I rest and trust as I await your sacred, spontaneous combustion. Amen.

In Awe of Resilience

⌐ The delicate and fragile nature of humans is astonishing! They are susceptible to illness, disease, and injury. They also are robust and hardy, endowed with amazing powers of healing that permeate body, mind, and spirit. Have you wondered or even asked your patients, "How did you get through that ordeal?" This question actually is about yourself as you consider, "Could I handle what they faced?" The answer to that question is, "Yes, you can handle life's challenges." You can face life's difficult moments, thanks to the love of your family, the encouragement of your friends, the support of your colleagues, and the hope and trust grounded in your spirituality. There is a sacred staff upon which you lean that helps you walk and not faint. The well from which you draw the waters of resiliency is deep.

Passion Care: A Reflection

⌐ Think about your present excitement as a healer. Are you feeling content at this time in your career? Do you find your work satisfying? Do high morale and spirits pervade your team? Are you eager to get to work?

It is important that you identify those factors creating and sustaining your enthusiasm. Once you identify these elements, you will be able to cultivate and protect them, more fully integrating them into your daily activities. Are there others on your team who you can approach and enlist in the effort to sustain these spirit-building aspects within the life of the team?

On the other hand, are you sensing that your present situation is losing its appeal to you? Do you have to force yourself to show up at work? Do you feel tired and uninspired? Find a time when you can think about what is going on. Conduct a self-assessment and a work-culture assessment. Sort out those dynamics, interactions, and experiences that are energy drainers, the ones that dampen your spirits.

Do you see ways to engage those components with the goal of changing or eliminating them for your own good and for the good of your colleagues? How will you go about seeking this change? Who can you enlist as a colleague in these efforts?

Purpose Is a Multifaceted Jewel

⌐ Your life is purposeful. Reflect on the myriad purposes gracing your life. If you are married, one of your purposes is to be a loving and encouraging partner. If you are a parent, you have the purpose of being a nurturing and caring parent. With your friends, your purpose is to be trustworthy. As you work with your patients, your purpose is to be a compassionate and competent healer. As a human, your purpose is to live the life given to you as fully as possible in harmony and beauty with your neighbors and with creation. Marvel at the many purposes that add color and depth to your life, each contributing to your life's fullness and blessedness. Remember, your purpose to be a health care professional is one of many.

CHAPTER II

Offer Kindness and Humility

HEALTH CARE is a performance-based world. Status and esteem are based on your outcomes and productivity. However, your performance is what you do, not who you are. Be mindful of the distinction. The spiritual experience of the Transcendent Source of Life discloses to you that you are valued in and of yourself. Your experience of being valued for who you are rather than what you do is one of Grace.

This experience with the Transcendent Source of Life evokes a sense of humility. This humility arises from the realization that all creation is a gift. In particular, your life is a gift. How amazing it is that you are alive and that you possess the qualities and characteristics that particularize you! You certainly helped shape yourself through education and training. However, the raw material you used in that shaping was given to you as a gift, the cause of humble gratitude. Humility permits you to be kind and gentle with yourself and to offer kindness to others. We all have our strengths and our limitations.

The power of performance to define who you are is signaled by your sense of inadequacy. Inadequacy will stir up thoughts and feelings of apprehension about your abilities and ultimately about yourself. You may tend to view yourself as not good enough or as one who does not belong in health care.

The key is for you to maintain a sense of balance at those times when your performance is not up to your usual standards or when a particular patient does not respond as well as hoped. Your experience of Grace is invaluable in sustaining that balance; it holds back the tidewaters of inadequacy that occasionally rise within you. It also enables you to extend kindness to others as well as yourself.

GRANT AND TED'S STORY: AT THE END OF BEING ON CALL IN THE HOSPITAL

Night call can find you flying all over the hospital, responding to this page, and then to another page. You have no time to rest, and you fuel up on coffee and nibbles as best you can. When the end of your call approaches, you begin to watch the clock, counting the minutes when your relief arrives, and you can turn over the pager to your colleague.

On this particular night, Grant's pager never seemed to stop beeping! Page came on top of page. He was drained physically and emotionally. At 0700, his relief still had not arrived to take the pager. Grant found himself growing increasingly irritated that Ted was late—again! He knew it was too much to ask for Ted to arrive at 0645 so that Grant could review the events of the night and hand-off the pager. Surely, Grant thought, Ted would have the decency to show up at 0700, the start of his on call rotation.

Finally, at 0718, Ted paged Grant. Grant met Ted at the nurses' station. Ted simply said, "Hi—how did it go?" Not one word of apology or explanation regarding his tardiness. Grant told Ted in no uncertain terms how angry he was at Ted's inconsiderate and unprofessional conduct. Curtly, Grant briefed Ted on the calls of the night, and turned and walked away from Ted. Grant could feel his cheeks flush and the hair stand on the back of his neck. He was mad!

Since Ted and Grant were colleagues, their paths crossed often. In the ensuing days, neither one of them spoke about that night. They exchanged only the minimum acknowledgments. As time passed, Grant grew uncomfortable with the rift he had created, and with his own inner stirrings. He realized that he had not inquired about what made Ted late that night— he only assumed that "once again" Ted was being inconsiderate and nonchalant. He knew that he was tired at the end of his call, and that he handled his exasperation with Ted poorly. Certainly he was not pleased with Ted. More importantly, Grant was disappointed in himself.

One day, the two of them happened onto each other on the floor. After exchanging stilted greetings, Grant asked Ted if they could talk. "Sure," replied Ted. Grant stated that he wanted to revisit their interaction when Ted came on call to relieve Grant. Grant acknowledged that he did not inquire about what made Ted late and that his speech was harsh. He stated that he regretted that conversation and would like to apologize and get back on better terms with Ted. Grant waited to see how Ted would reply. Ted looked at Grant and said . . .

The conclusion to the conversation between Grant and Ted is purposely omitted. There is always the uncertainty of how another person will respond to your offer of forgiveness or your request to be forgiven. What matters in the above experience is that Grant reached the point where he saw the benefit to him and to Ted in requesting forgiveness. Hopefully, Ted accepted Grant's request to be forgiven. If not, Grant at least could take comfort in his effort to achieve reconciliation.

As the Christian scripture wisely says, "The eye cannot say to the hand, 'I have no need of you,' nor again the head to the feet, 'I have no need of you.'" Humility sees how all things work together to care for the patient. Patient care requires numerous hands. Some hands directly touch the patient. Other hands indirectly touch the patient. Humility respects all the hands, not just one's own, that make patient care possible. Consider the invaluable contribution of the hands of the housekeepers.

Praise the Housekeepers: An Ounce of Prevention Is Worth a Pound of Cure

Infection control is one of a hospital's top priorities. All the staff and team members follow infection control and prevention practices, protocols, and procedures. Housekeeping operates at a fairly inconspicuous level in a hospital. Yet, housekeepers play a key role in the fight against infection. When a patient's room is vacated, that room has to be cleaned and prepared for the next patient—"turned around." Such preparation includes wiping down and cleaning all the surfaces in the room. The mattress, bed rail, counters, fixtures, chairs, bedside tables, and the bathroom all are cleaned and wiped down. Only after a thorough preparation is the new patient admitted into that room. It is not an exaggeration to say that housekeepers are on the front line in the battle against infection.

This example of how housekeepers cooperate with others to combat infection demonstrates that much of what you and your colleagues do is one piece of a much larger picture. Humility is the realization that you have a place—a distinct role—in patient care. Your place is invaluable, no matter what role you play. You may do the surgery. You may be the one who diagnosed the patient. You may be the one who stocks the supply room or refills the medications cart. You may sterilize the instruments or clean the room. You may repair the monitors, instruments, or devices so that they function and perform flawlessly. You may start the IV. You may mix the contents of the bolus. You may deliver linens to the floor. You may clean the halls and waiting rooms. You may work in the kitchen or be the one who plans the meal appropriate to this patient. You may pray with the patient and family.

Humility is an inward and outward realization. The inward realization is the awareness of the contribution you make. It is the realization of how you fit into the circle of care surrounding the patient. Humility entails respecting and honoring the difference you make. It is safe to say that humility is self-respect.

The outward realization of humility is your appreciation for all the others who, like you, play vital roles in patient care. Other members of the team may have more credentials or education, or they may have fewer qualifications and training. They may make a higher or lower salary than you. Their authority may be greater or lesser than yours. Such considerations have no bearing on the contribution they make to patient care.

Actually, all such considerations of "Who is more important?" are insignificant in the grand scheme of patient care. Such thinking is detrimental to the strength of the health care team. Gone unchecked, such evaluative thinking can disrupt the team's homeostasis, causing various unwelcome symptoms to appear— jealousy, envy, animosity, disrespect, and even rifts. The health of the health care team itself requires respect and appreciation. Each person on the team needs the other person in order to provide safe, quality, and compassionate care. Humility is this realization and appreciation of interdependence.

Humility further consists of being open to the insights, suggestions, and recommendations of other members of the health care team regarding "doing what is good" for the patient. Humility enables you to listen to your colleagues and to consider their insights and comments. Drawing on their experience and training, your colleagues may disagree with the patient care approach you propose. In such instances, what matters is not *who* is right, but *what* is right.

You as a healer have an appropriate commitment to accuracy and to being right in terms of diagnosis, prognosis, and treatment/intervention. In the best of worlds, these two positions of "being right" and "doing good" work hand in hand. They are two sides of the same coin. Being right is not about winning an argument or even proving the flawed thinking of a colleague. It is about benefiting the patient.

A spectacular instance of experiencing interdependence and humility is when all the hospital's electrical power was lost. This crisis affected everyone in the hospital. Consider this example of humility and interdependence.

Everyone Matters: Nothing Like a Power Outage to Put Things in Perspective!

Up to the moment of the power failure, the hospital was going about its business. Surgeries were underway. CAT scans, X-ray machines, lights, soft drink machines, and respirators were working. Then, suddenly, the lights went out, darkening surgery suites, waiting rooms, and patient rooms. Ventilators were silenced. The screens of monitors went blank. Elevators were immobilized. Emergency procedures and protocols are rehearsed in drills to prepare for emergencies. In this instance, it was not a drill: the power outage was real! Both the primary and back-up sources of power failed.

People moved into action. Overhead announcements began. Flashlights were broken out to provide illumination. All respirator-dependent patients were "bagged," receiving each breath by the hands of a staff member squeezing a hand-compressed bag ventilator. The building and grounds team moved into high gear. The power company was promptly notified. In short order, the hospital's power was restored. Everyone breathed a sigh of relief and of gratitude!

Such emergencies can only be managed by the combined efforts of many teams and individuals. Everyone plays an indispensable role in responding to an emergency. Emergencies are an opportunity to witness how your team worked hand in hand with other teams to manage the crisis. This realization is one of pride, as well as humility. The pride is in your personal and your team's combined efforts: you did well and the team did well. Humility comes from the appreciation of how many others were required to meet this emergency.

PRAYERS, MEDITATIONS, AND REFLECTIONS

A Wake-Up Call

Sacred Spirit, I took an unnecessary risk with a patient today by being cocky. I know better. I put myself above the patient. One of my colleagues told me later, "You were courting disaster today buddy and dodged a bullet. Better thank your lucky stars." Those words shook me to the core. What was I thinking? I am so grateful that things turned out as well as they did, especially for the patient. May this "near-miss" ever accompany and guide me, a friend who constantly reminds me to be humble, to be cautious, and to check with others. Thank you for the wake-up call. Amen.

Confidence Counts

It is one thing to be confident and another to be conceited. I have worked hard to build up my confidence. My confidence is based upon my successful completion of the many requirements to become a healer. Confidence gives me the freedom to continue to learn so that my confidence is increased. Nothing stays the same. For me to stay current means that I learn new approaches and techniques.

In contrast, conceit is one face of fear. Conceit will blind me to my learning edges. It will deafen my ears to the announcement of new breakthroughs and developments. The safeguard from conceit is humility. Humility protects my confidence, keeps it in perspective and in proportion. I am confident enough to say in all humility that "I know what I do not know."

Without My Help, Sometimes Things Fall into Place

Creator, help me to embrace humility. There are moments in patient care when the right person is in the right place at the right time. I have nothing to do with their presence when the patient needed help. It may be a moment when a tech or an aide is walking down the hall and, realizing a patient is in distress, immediately alerts the clinicians.

Maybe a chaplain is visiting the patient and family when the patient begins a rapid decline and beckons the nurse. How do these things happen? I am not always the one who directs and oversees the care of the patient. There are these moments when good things happen for patients without any of my assistance. I am humbled by and grateful for this mystery that sometimes good things happen. Amen.

A Prayer of Humble Thanksgiving

Mysterious Source of Sacred Stillness, I need your steadying presence. Never in my career have I had available the means to save a life and had my hands tied. We did our best to tell her of the considerable risk—a potentially fatal risk—facing her without a simple and routine intervention that could remove the threat to her life. Her mind was set: she declined what would easily save her life.

And so, we stood by as witnesses to her death. It was agony for all of us—nurses, physicians, chaplains. Tears were shed as we watched her life slip away. My heart is broken. As I recover from the pain and anguish of this event, help me find solace. I did adhere to the patient's wishes. As a healer, I need to know that somehow I helped this patient, as painful as it was for me. The help that meant the most to this patient was my honoring her wishes. In doing so, I served her.

May this case prepare me for countless future patient care moments—moments where what I do that matters is to abide by the preferences of the patient. Grant me the gift of being heartened and consoled by doing what the patient wants. Amen.

Humility's Helping Hand

My patients can count on me. I am dependable. I am able to work independently, make my own assessments, devise my own treatments, apply my own bandages, administer medications, and be a compassionate, healing presence.

At the same time, I am keenly aware of my scope of practice. I know enough to ask for a consult or help. I know enough to refer a patient. I have the independence to ask a colleague, or my supervisor, for their advice or suggestions. I am respected for this trait. People know that I am not a bull in a china shop, a lone ranger, or some fool who rushes in where angels fear to tread. Yes, I am independent. I am counted on to do what is required and expected of me. Simultaneously, humility has taught me that everybody needs an extra hand, another set of eyes, another mind fairly frequently.

Standing in Humility's Sacred Presence

Call to mind a time when you experienced firsthand the presence of humility. Think about a respected teacher, mentor, or peer. Remember a moment when you witnessed his or her humility and, in that moment, stood in the healing presence, the sacred presence, of humility.

Make the memory as detailed as possible—sights, sounds, smells, time, light, colors, words, expressions, attire, and actions. Ease yourself into that memory, and ask:

▸ What am I thinking, sensing, and feeling in this moment?

▸ What healing insights are coming to me?

▸ How may I apply these healing insights to the aches of my body, mind, and spirit?

Meditation Starters for Humility

▤ I am not of my own making. I did not ask to be born at this time, to these parents, in this nation, as a member of this race, with these traits, with these strengths, with these weaknesses. Nonetheless, I was beckoned here.

> ▸ What is my destiny?
> ▸ How does my destiny depend on others?
> ▸ How does the destiny of others depend on me?

Reflections of Myself

▤ When I am so offended by the cocky attitude of someone, their arrogance and bloated sense of self-importance, I wonder what about that person resembles me. What reflection of myself do I behold in the mirror of that person? How am I able to see the speck in another's eye, yet be oblivious to the plank in my own eye?

Ironically, my incensed attitude, if not outright disgust at their self-adoration, is in itself a form of pride! My reaction to that other person's inflated pride is a message to me and about me.

Actually, my reaction is an invitation. The invitation is for me to look inward at my own heart and soul. Bit by bit, I use what humility I possess to face honestly my infatuation with myself and view myself more realistically. I do possess certain aptitudes and realize that there are skills and knowledge I do not possess. (I think that's why healers make referrals or ask for a consultation.) I am a person of integrity. I have a sense of humor. I am valued, but I am not indispensable.

The Health Found in Humility

I cannot sustain this pace. I am spent—mentally, physically, emotionally, and spiritually. My home life is on the rocks. My circle of friends is dwindling. My colleagues are more distant, more formal, a little cooler toward me. No wonder: I am so important—at least in my head—that I have little patience for such things as time with my beloved, with my children, with my friends. I am in so much pain—I hide it. I am scared.

I am teetering on the brink of employing ill-advised methods to keep up this façade and this pace, to dampen this pain, to boost my energy. I can't play God anymore. I thought that I wanted to be God, and that I could actually be God. I have to liberate myself from this pride-driven obsession before it is too late. Two paths stand clearly before me. One path is pride. Its destination is ruin. One path is humility. Its destination is fulfillment.

Humility and Joy

What an upper! Our team was outstanding! Everybody did his or her part. We succeeded. It was tremendous—unbelievable. It was like we were reading each other's minds. We didn't have to ask: we knew. We anticipated what was next and were ready for it. It was a thing to behold—pieces falling into place as though choreographed, as though orchestrated—amazing! What a rare moment.

We don't need any award or recognition. We know in our hearts and souls what happened today is wonderful—the right people in the right place at the right time doing the right thing. It really is humbling when you think about it. It was the accomplishment of a team, a group, a system. I am hard pressed to say which feels better—the accomplishments of my own hand or the accomplishment of the team. I find that belonging to a team, and doing my part, is actually more satisfying. It connected us, united us, and bound us together so that the sum was greater than the parts. Can't beat that!

A Bragger's Confession

Holy One, have mercy on me, a bragger! Today I took most of the credit for pulling a patient through a critical time. I barely acknowledged the contributions made by the rest of the team, talking about what "I" did, rather than what "we" did. Please forgive me. Grant me the courage to apologize to those who helped care for this patient. I pray that they are able to forgive me. I know that I cannot undo the hurt my words inflicted. My future words and actions are my only hope for healing in this complicated web of my own making. Amen.

In Search of Self-Forgiveness

Think on this: you are forgiven—this sense is rooted in your experience of the Transcendent Source of Life. In that experience you are aware that you—imperfections, shortcomings, and all—are valued and deemed worthy. God forgives you. Your colleague forgives you. Somehow, you cannot accept the forgiveness offered you. You cannot forgive yourself. Is it possible that your inability to accept forgiveness reveals that you are holding yourself to higher standards and expectations that those of your friends and those of the Transcendent Source of Life?

What keeps you from accepting the forgiveness offered to you? Humility offers you the path to forgiveness. Humility frees you from your preoccupation with being perfect, and permits you to be gentle and kind to your true self, the one that like other humans is limited and imperfect. There is well-being in being able to say to yourself and to others, "Yes, I messed up—thanks for your understanding and forgiveness." Try taking two pills of humility and see if you feel better in the morning.

CHAPTER 12

Express Encouragement, Gratitude, and Humor

WITH ALL ITS pressures, frustrations, and problems, you are grateful to be a participant in healing. You truly are blessed. You have the privilege of being with people at some of the most trying times in their lives. They welcome you into their lives without hesitation. Patients explicitly trust you as being committed to their well-being. You are making a difference in the lives of patients and families. Your work is profoundly meaningful. You tell yourself every so often, "Wow—I am so lucky!" There are plenty of other moments when opposite thoughts come to mind: thoughts of all that is wrong with your job or with health care. Be that as it may, those moments are unable to surmount your basic and pervasive attitude of gratitude.

Gratitude, then, is your basic disposition. It exists apart from external events and circumstances. You are able to "be thankful in all circumstances," as the Apostle Paul, a teacher of long ago, encouraged early Christians to be. Such gratitude is far from flippant. It is not blind to the current realities. It is not looking at life with rose-colored glasses. To the contrary, in your spirituality, gratitude is a core disposition that is keenly aware of the tragic and hostile in life. Gratitude beholds, embraces, and takes in the sorrow and hurt of the present condition, possessing the power to keep you grateful in life's most bleak situations. When the storms of life roar and unleash the furies against you, your patients and their families, or your colleagues, it is your gratitude that sustains and carries you. Given all that is wrong, unjust, tragic, and sorrowful, your gratitude encourages and empowers you. It is precisely in these moments of trial that your ability to be grateful upholds and shelters you and those about you.

Take a moment to enter the world of the following event.

Ron's Story: Gratitude When Efforts Are Unsuccessful

Ron had a history of respiratory ailments, from childhood into his adult years. He had been admitted to the hospital to be treated for the flu. The team placed Ron on a medical/surgical floor where his recovery was coming along well. The health care team expected that he would be discharged in the next few days.

Unexpectedly, sometime in the late evening, Ron went into respiratory arrest. A code blue was called, and that team arrived promptly. Working cooperatively and effectively, the team began its efforts to recover the patient's respiration. They were hopeful, in part because of their experience and skill and in part because of the age and status of the patient. They inserted tubes, established lines, began medications, and started chest compressions.

Early on, it was clear that Ron was in serious distress. His breathing simply would not respond to their efforts. The physician overseeing the code ordered new interventions. These, too, proved ineffective. At last, as it was clear that Ron was not going to be resuscitated, the physician called the code. The team was saddened and discouraged, with many of them puzzled by their inability to save this patient. He had a wife and children.

As the team members went about cleaning up the room, the physician asked for their attention. When they stopped what they were doing and looked at the physician, he simply stated: "I thank each and every one of you for what you did tonight. We worked well as a team. We did our best for this patient. I know the outcome is painful. Please know I am grateful for what you did tonight." His few words of gratitude eased the hearts, souls, and minds of the team. Those words of gratitude were a gift in the midst of great sorrow and disappointment.

At its core, this clinical episode is sad. A patient unexpectedly stopped breathing, and nothing the code blue team attempted succeeded in restoring his breathing. Yet, in the very center of this tragedy, the physician was able to be grateful. The physician felt the pain and disappointment of the team. In a moment, the physician would be talking with Ron's family and knew fully that they would be grief stricken to learn of their loved one's death. Nonetheless, in that room where the team had labored mightily in behalf of the patient, the physician saw reason to be grateful. This ability to experience gratitude, and to communicate that gratitude to others, meant a great deal to everyone involved in this valiant effort to save a patient.

Gratitude is a key daily spiritual practice. This spiritual discipline may well begin when you awaken. You have been called from sleep to live this particular day. You had a bed upon which to rest, a roof under which to sleep, blankets for warmth, loved ones present with you. Now, upon waking, you receive the gift of yet another day. It's not just any day, but this particular and precious day—a day with its awaiting gifts, challenges, and opportunities—all beckoning you.

As the day unfolds, you are able to continue your gratitude exercises as you give thanks for your eyes, ears, legs, hands, and mind. You have multiple instances to be grateful for the instruments and medicines of healing, for the collaboration of your colleagues, for patients and families entrusted into your care and keeping, and for the blessing of being granted the gift of bringing health and healing to others.

ENCOURAGEMENT: THE POWER OF APPRECIATION

You know all too well that health care is frequently a thankless undertaking. You and your team may think: "I am supposed to be doing my job. This is my responsibility. I am merely doing what is required—why should I expect to be thanked?" You have ethical, legal, and organizational obligations to do your particular task. You are fulfilling the responsibilities of your particular role. All of this is true. However, none of the above eliminates the significance of saying thank you or for showing appreciation to another person for their efforts. Appreciation—whether it is expressed by patients, families, managers, or senior leaders—has the all-important power to encourage you and your colleagues.

Words of appreciation may be rare in health care. Simple phrases like "thank you," "you did a good job," or "I do not take your consistent performance for granted" are few and far between. Instead of words of appreciation, the conversation is likely to be about targets that are to be met. These targets are set for your team and for you. While there is a celebration and recognition when targets are achieved, the pressure to achieve is unrelenting. Any success is quickly replaced with new—and even higher and more demanding—goals. Rarely is appreciation expressed for your character, your enthusiasm, your positive outlook, your trustworthiness, your consistently good work, or your dependability.

Healers, like others, certainly work to earn their salary—money matters. However, it is widely known that a good salary is not enough to retain staff or improve staff/employee satisfaction. Healers do not live by salary alone, but by words of appreciation.

Additionally, you and your colleagues are highly motivated individuals. Your passion as a healer is to help others. You are deeply committed to human well-being. You carry your internal measures of competency and success and often know that you and your team performed well. This self-appreciation of your own commitment and your inner awareness of the quality of your care are invaluable. However, this inner appreciation of your personal attributes requires the accompanying recognition experienced in the words and actions of gratitude from patients, families, colleagues, and administrators.

Here is an instance that captures the power of an encouraging and simple thank you.

GIVING THANKS: THE GIFT OF GRATITUDE

Hospital switchboard operators are the communication hub of the hospital. Calls come in from family members, friends of the patients, physicians, other affiliated hospitals within the system, community hospitals, the fire department, law enforcement, administrators and senior leaders, various branches of the military, and others. Switchboard operators handle all the emergency signals, such as code blues and internal and external disaster situations (for example, fire, loss of power, bad weather, bomb threat, mass casualties, etc.). They take calls from people who are sad, confused, or angry. Often, this team is under quite a bit of pressure, experiencing high levels of stress.

All this activity occurs in a small area, far removed from the hubbub of the hospital units and floors. Though out of sight, this team functions 24-7, playing a critical, if unseen, role in patient care and safety. Words of gratitude to them are few and far between.

On some occasions, this team helps alert a chaplain of an urgent request from the clinical team. Their efforts include activating the chaplain's pager as well as sending an overhead announcement that the on-call chaplain is needed immediately. With their efforts, the operators contribute to patient and family care as well as staff support.

One of the practices of the chaplains as they report for their on-call shift is to stop by the switchboard office, as the on-call pager permits. Routinely, the chaplains enter the switchboard area and move from operator to operator saying in so many words, "Thanks for all you do." Smiles appear on the faces of the operators. In response, they say, "You are welcome—and thanks for what you do." More specifically, the chaplains express their gratitude for the efforts made by the operators to ensure a prompt response by the chaplains and others to an urgent situation. They acknowledge the invaluable role played by the switchboard team in patient and family care and staff support.

When the chaplains leave the switchboard area, smiles linger on the operators' faces. A brief exchange that thanked them and acknowledged their importance was a great moral booster. Gratitude matters.

This one example demonstrates how expressions of gratitude have the power to encourage. Words of appreciation are energizing. Spirits are lifted by a simple thank you. Expressions of appreciation from patients and families vary, influenced by the patient's and family's unique history and outlook. Many of your patients and their families are direct with their appreciation for what you have done. Some of your patients and families say thank you every so often. You know those patients and families who are unlikely to ever express words of gratitude. Those appreciative patients are the ones who feed your soul.

With your colleagues and leaders, the situation is a bit different. Compliments from a peer are honored, in as much as such expressions are based on a respect for the challenge you met and the competencies required of you to respond successfully to that challenge. Compliments from leaders are honored as well, as they signal recognition for the quality of your patient care. A simple thank you from a leader acknowledges and affirms your integrity and abilities as a healer, one who consistently provides quality care in the midst of the trying, tiring, and stressful world of health care.

Earlier, I said that your gratitude radiates, bringing light and warmth to others. Gratitude is another manifestation of the interdependence of life. Your level of gratitude affects your colleagues and your patients. Expressions of gratitude from leaders ripple throughout a team. Words of appreciation from your patients and families lift your spirits and touch your heart. Appreciation is mutual: it is reciprocal. Appreciation blesses the giver and the recipient.

Humor: Laughter as a Healing Power

Healers need a sense of humor. Perhaps the public at large is most familiar with the healer's professional outward persona. Your attire—smocks, laboratory coats, stethoscopes, scrubs, scissors, uniforms, cargo pants, and masks—communicate the image of a person who is serious, knowledgeable, deliberate, and thoughtful. More often than not, you are treated with formality, deference, and respect. There are exceptions, of course, where a bit more respect and cooperation, and less curtness and antagonism, would be welcome!

Health care is serious—no doubt about it. There is a lot at stake in providing patient care. It is important that you and your colleagues be focused and disciplined. There is no margin for error. Accuracy is imperative. Patient assessment and diagnosis need to be precise, as they are the foundation for safe treatment and excellent care. Standards of care, procedures, protocols, and policies provide the parameters for the provision of care.

However, humor is alive and well in health care! Actually, humor is *critical* in such a serious setting as health care. Humor relieves stress and pressure. It provides a bit of play and lightness. Humor is imperative if someone wants to have a career in health care. Perhaps humor needs to be part of the screening process for those seeking to enter health care. If that were the case, applicants who demonstrate a sense of humor would move forward in the application process, while those who possess little or no humor would be encouraged to consider other career options.

Humor is the ability to laugh, first and foremost, at yourself. You know your peculiarities and idiosyncrasies better than anyone else—although your colleagues have a pretty good idea! Chuckling at yourself is healthier than berating yourself. You will show up at work with shaving cream in your ear or toothpaste in the corner of your mouth. Your zipper will not be completely closed, or you will have toilet paper stuck to your shoe. One day, you may have on socks that do not match—or even mismatching shoes! The ability to smile while saying—silently or out loud—"Gee—how did I do that?!" is far and away preferable to giving yourself a dressing down of "What was I thinking?!" Criticism is alive and well. It does not need your help to thrive. Chuckles and smiles are able to flourish given proper nourishment. Being able to laugh at yourself strengthens your resiliency and helps you maintain your humility.

It is important to have the ability to laugh at situations as well. The humor may be at hand in the moment, with smiles and laughter occurring spontaneously when you make a slip of the tongue or ask others to help you find your glasses while they are hanging around your neck. At other times, the situation does not strike you as funny. You may be frustrated or embarrassed that your pen ran out of ink while you were making notes in the patient's chart. You may be in the midst of an oration against one of the new policies just introduced by administration, only to have one of the senior leaders standing nearby, out of sight but within earshot. It may take a bit of reflection and time for you to be able to look back and smile at these and other countless situations. There is a time to laugh and a time not to laugh.

Humor is also a group activity. Humor creates bonds and connections among and between people. Your ability to join your colleagues in a good laugh—whether at the nurses' station or in the break room—communicates that you are one of them. Stories circulate in the hospital or up on the floors. Many of these stories are funny and bring a laugh every time they are recounted. Yarns and folklore are widespread, existing among teams and on floors and units.

These tales begin with:

▸ "Do you remember the time when . . . ?"
▸ "Remember that patient in Room 333 . . . ?"
▸ "Were you there when Joe or Jane forgot . . . ?"
▸ "I will always remember what happened that morning when one of our senior leaders was rounding on the floor because . . . "
▸ "You should have been here when we saw a patient walking down the hall with the back of his/her gown wide open!"

Your interactions with patients and families also offer you opportunities for smiles and laughs. Patients and families are capable of wit. Sometimes they make an off-handed joke about some event in the news. Or they may relate some funny incident in their life or family. You know those patients who possess an enduring sense of humor. They draw upon that humor as a reservoir of courage and resolve during the course of their illness. In most circumstances, they are able to interject humor with witty one-liners or quips. What they are doing is inviting you to join them in a smile, a laugh, or a chuckle—accept their invitation! Smiling with your patients strengthens your relationship and contributes to their well-being (and yours as well!).

CHARLEY'S STORY: WHEN DRESS CODES ARE SECONDARY TO PATIENT CARE

Charley was a physician who was admitted to the hospital where he worked. He was well-known among the health care team. One day, a code blue was announced on his floor. Without a second thought, Charley jumped out of bed and headed toward the scene of the code blue—that's what physicians do. As he raced down the hall, the back of his gown was wide open, flapping with every step—a sight beheld by staff and visitors!

After the code ended successfully, the health care team provided him another gown to cover his backside as he returned to his room. In the days following, this story was told and retold with admiration—and with humor!

What funny stories cause you to chuckle? Think back to the days of your education and training. What humorous pieces of folklore did you hear about otherwise respected colleagues? What were your humorous interactions? These stories are a breath of fresh air. Treasure them—especially the ones involving you! Your ability to tell funny stories about yourself is a good sign of your own well-being.

PRAYERS, MEDITATIONS, AND REFLECTIONS

Count Your Blessings

You move in a problem-focused and solution-seeking environment. This focus can lead to seeing only what is wrong and needs fixing. Gratitude offers you a wider horizon.

Give yourself time each day to review what fills you with gratitude. Make a mental or written list of the simple things for which you are grateful—things you might take for granted or which are pushed out of mind by the pace of the day. For instance, you are alive (you did not ask to be alive—to be this person in this place at this time). This day awaits you, filled with adventure. The sun came up. You are breathing (oxygen is provided free of charge!). You see and hear (sights and sounds surround you). You bathe and clothe yourself—oh, how your skin loves the touch of water and cloth! You have food and shelter. Water and electricity are at your fingertips. You have knowledge and skills. There are people you love, and who love you (name them, see their faces, hear their voices, feel their touch).

Keep going—ponder those simple gifts and wonders for which you are grateful. During your day, gratitude can help maintain your perspective about what matters and preserve your priorities in life.

Encouragement's Life-Giving Water

O Holy One, my soul is parched, thirsty for an encouraging word. Work has turned into a barren wasteland. Every day, I am exposed to expectation's soul-drying heat. My spirit is dehydrated. People are as hard as rocks. Breach the dams that hold captive the thirst-slaking words of appreciation. Open the floodgates of the soul-hydrating words of gratitude. May I, in turn, be a spring from which flows words of appreciation. In my words and by my actions may I be a well of life-giving water where others may drink to their heart's satisfaction. Amen.

In Praise of Humor

Divine One, what a hoot that you saw fit to create us as creatures whose well-being requires good laughs on a daily basis. Since we are made in your image, you must have some sense of humor. We see your playfulness as leaves twirl and dance in the wind, as squirrels chase one another around the trunk of a tree, and as the moon dares to eclipse mighty Mr. Sun's light! Thank you for jokes, quips, irony, puns, and parody! Thank you for the unsuspecting angels who sprinkle humor through our day, lifting our spirits, spreading smiles across our faces, and igniting a twinkle in our eyes. Amen.

Afterword

ORDINARILY, books end with a conclusion. This book now reaches the point of continuation. There really are few conclusions in life. On the surface, it seems that life has stops and starts, or starts and stops. Upon closer examination, each ending serves as the beginning of the next step, such as they both blend and merge into a continuous flow. If we were to look at walking, we might say that the walk ends with the stride of the left foot. In actuality, the planting of the left foot serves as the basis from which the right foot lifts, swings, and plants, accomplishing the next step. And so this movement we call walking continues— planting, swinging, lifting, planting, swinging, and lifting.

Your journey continues. Our conversation, to change images from that of walking, is one of listening and speaking. Dialogue is that circular dance of listening, then speaking. You and I have conversed about healing. I hope that I have listened well to you. I hope as well that what I have spoken addresses the heart of the matter and, more importantly, *your* heart.

May you be blessed in experiencing that in healing, you are healed. Yours is a sacred constellation, where science, humanity, the tangible, and the intangible orbit and swirl. Stay amazed!

About the Author

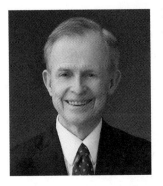 Rev. Dr. William E. Dorman was the director of chaplaincy services for the largest integrated health care system in New Mexico, Presbyterian Healthcare Services, where he was invited to be the only nonclinical member of the professional standards review committee. He left Presbyterian Healthcare Services after eighteen years to become the bereavement coordinator for Gentiva Hospice in Albuquerque, New Mexico, where he served bereaved family members and coached and supported members of the hospice team.

Presently, Rev. Dr. Dorman is an adult military family life counselor at the Kirtland Air Force Base in Albuquerque. He and his colleagues provide help with such matters as resiliency, coping skills, anger management, grief and loss, parenting, and relationship challenges (predeployment, reintegration, postdeployment).

Rev. Dr. Dorman has spoken in multiple settings across the years to physicians, nurses, civic clubs, employee groups, city employees, committees, nursing students, faith groups, and boards. He has presented on the benefit of spirituality to health to varied audiences, such as at Grand Rounds, a group for physicians; at the annual conference of the Association of Professional Chaplains; and at the annual Spirituality and Health Conference, where he has been one of the main presenters and a panel respondent.

Dorman is theologically educated and clinically trained. He earned his doctor of ministry and master of divinity degrees from Vanderbilt University Divinity School. He is a licensed marriage and family therapist, a board certified chaplain (Association of Professional Chaplains), an International Critical Incident Stress Foundation (ICISF) Approved Instructor for individual and peer crisis intervention as well as group crisis intervention. He is also a certified clinical bioethicist, trained at the University of Washington School of Medicine. He received additional training at the Kennedy Institute of Ethics at Georgetown University.

In February 2010, Rev. Dr. Dorman was a visiting scholar at the California Pacific Medical Center in the Program of Medicine and Human Values. At that center, he worked with Dr. Al Jonsen, PhD, concentrating on the bioethical issues related to intensive care unit patients.